The

MODERN WITCH'S

GUIDE

to

Magickal Self-Care

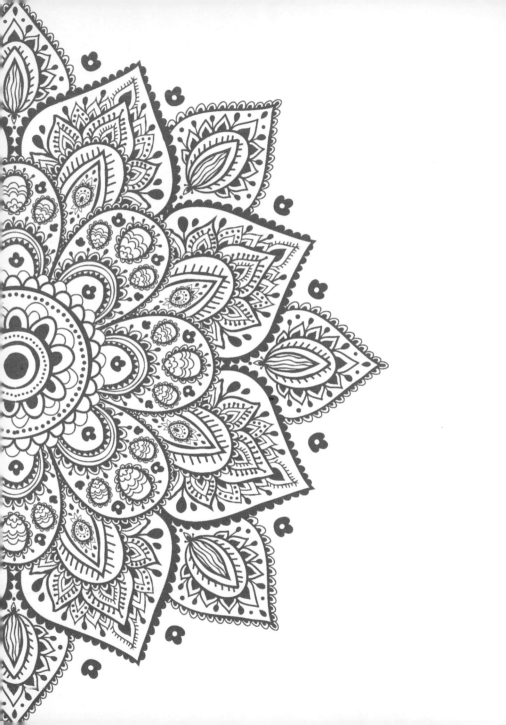

The
MODERN WITCH'S GUIDE
to
Magickal Self-Care

36 SUSTAINABLE RITUALS FOR NOURISHING YOUR MIND, BODY, AND INTUITION

TENAE STEWART

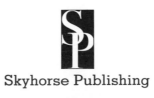

Skyhorse Publishing

Skyhorse Publishing books may be purchased in bulk at special discounts for sales promotion, corporate gifts, fund-raising, or educational purposes. Special editions can also be created to specifications. For details, contact the Special Sales Department, Skyhorse Publishing, 307 West 36th Street, 11th Floor, New York, NY 10018 or info@skyhorsepublishing.com.

Skyhorse® and Skyhorse Publishing® are registered trademarks of Skyhorse Publishing, Inc.®, a Delaware corporation.

Visit our website at www.skyhorsepublishing.com.

10 9 8 7 6 5 4 3

Library of Congress Cataloging-in-Publication Data is available on file.

Cover design by Daniel Brount
Cover photo by Chloe Marissa Wood

Print ISBN: 978-1-5107-5431-7
Ebook ISBN: 978-1-5107-5432-4

Printed in China

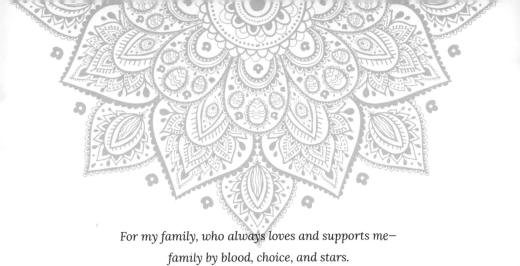

For my family, who always loves and supports me—
family by blood, choice, and stars.

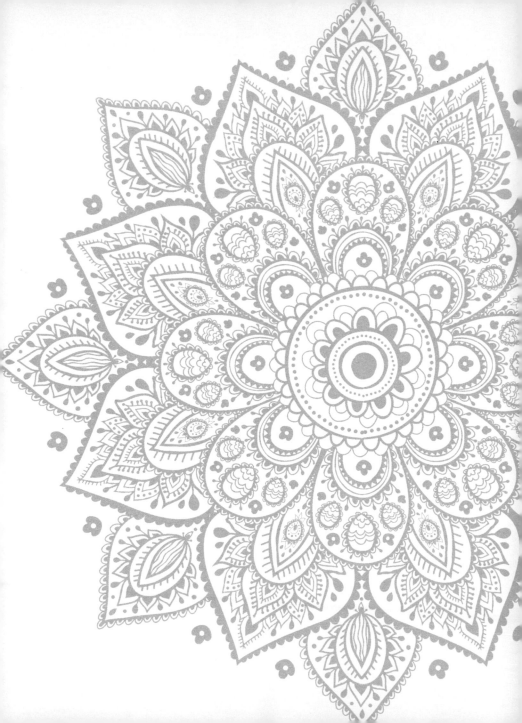

CONTENTS

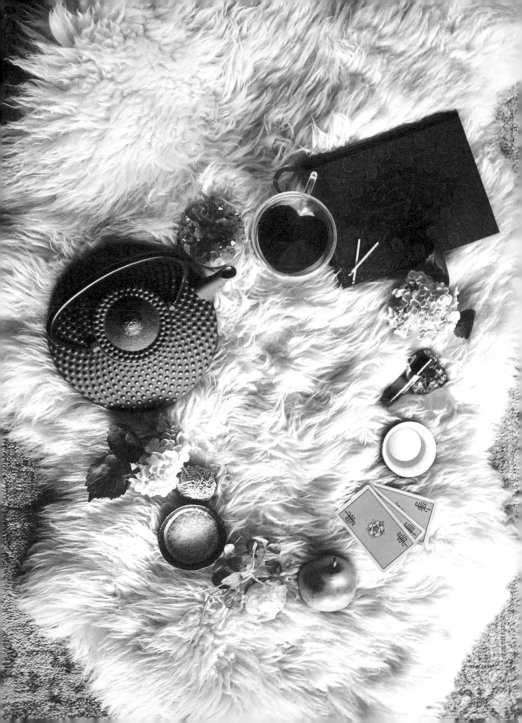

Preface

How do you define self-care?

Is it the day-to-day mundanities of meeting your physical needs? Is it the act of pampering yourself? Or is it a kind of deeper, spiritual fulfillment?

Self-care can look like each of these ideas, but truly caring for yourself requires a sacred combination of all three. The mundane, the luxurious, and the spiritual all have a place in your self-care practice, just as it is essential to honor the needs of the body, mind, and spirit equally.

If you have picked up this book, however, you might be wondering what witchcraft has to do with all of this. How do magic spells, pointy hats, and crooked wooden wands fit into a self-care practice? The short answer is that they don't, necessarily. Real modern witches might cast spells and occasionally wear pointy hats for the fun of it, but most of us practice a kind of witchcraft that is part self-development, part intuitive manifestation, and part nature-based paganism.

Certainly, there is an esoteric and metaphysical aspect to modern witchcraft which might look a bit different depending on the witch. Some read tarot cards, others follow the cycles of astrology and the moon phases, while still others worship ancient goddess archetypes or cast spells with candles and herbs. We will explore many of these different tools and techniques in this very book!

But witchcraft is about more than just the elements of magick, (the spiritual spelling with a "k" to differentiate from illusion and tricks), and the divine masculine and feminine around us. Modern witchcraft is also about tapping into your own intuition, learning to trust your instincts, and doing the shadow work on yourself so that you can grow, expand, and manifest the life that you want. Self-care is such an important part of that process of expansion, of stepping into your truest and most authentic potential. Even if you have all the right tools, you're doing all the journaling and shadow work, and you're making decisions based on your intuition, you can still fall victim to the pitfalls of a lack of self-care in your life. Burnout, overwhelm, stress-related illnesses, and the effects of an unhealthy lifestyle are just a few of the ailments that can overcome you when you aren't making self-care a priority.

This book is intended as a guide for women interested in deepening their self-care practice through witchcraft and magick. As both self-care and modern witchcraft become understood more and more as a part of the mainstream wellness culture, this conversation has made prioritizing the care of your mind, body, spirit, and intuition a core value of today's spiritual community. This community is putting greater stock in nourishing and sustainable self-care than ever before. This community is made up of readers like you who are getting in touch with your intuition and reclaiming the power in the word "witch," all while living out your normal, daily lives.

Witchcraft no longer needs to be a taboo topic with "scary" or "evil" associations. Self-care no longer needs to conjure images of lazing about in a bubble bath all day, while chores and obligations pile up. Witchcraft and self-care both have vital roles to play in the spiritual development of our age. By combining the elements of modern witchcraft with the mental health and wellness practices of self-care, you are creating a sacred space that honors all of your needs, not just those that are visible on the surface.

And that's exactly what we're going to do in this book!

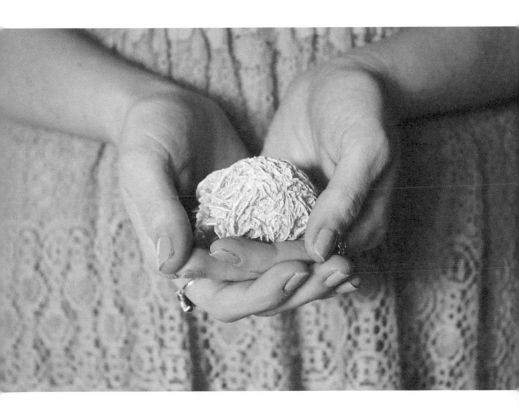

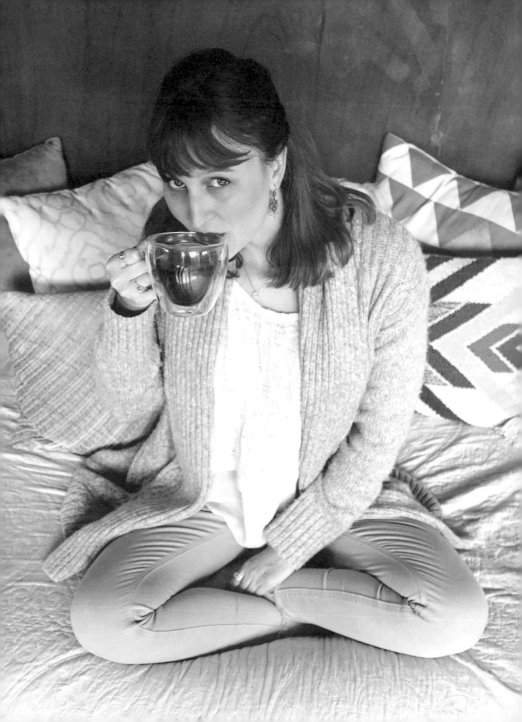

Chapter 1

WHAT DOES WITCHCRAFT HAVE TO DO WITH SELF-CARE?

As a professional witch and spiritual coach with my north node in Sagittarius in the fourth house of self-care, it is quite literally my soul purpose to explore my spirituality and to seek and share wisdom around the practice of creating sanctuary in which to care for my needs. Want to know what your soul purpose is and how to reach it?

Well, this book isn't going to magickally tell you that.

But don't be disappointed! What this book *is* going to tell you is how to identify your own unique needs, how to understand who you are at your core (including from an astrological perspective), and how to use the tools of witchcraft to create a support system of ritual and magick to fulfill those needs in the way that best suits you.

Because when you know who you are and what you need, the door to your soul purpose swings open and invites you in.

So what exactly does witchcraft have to do with self-care?

One of the first things I did when I began my journey as a witch was to celebrate the nature-based pagan practice of the sabbats. These eight seasonal holidays are based around the solstices, equinoxes, and the ancient fire festivals in between; along with following the moon cycle, these are what originally sparked my interest in witchcraft. The sabbats have incredible potential and power for connecting with nature, manifesting your dreams, and opening up your intuitive abilities. For a newbie witch, though, feeling connected to the sabbats, which are based on the ancient agricultural practices of planting, tending, and harvesting crops, can be a challenge.

Many new witches find themselves asking: What does any of this have to do with me? What do agricultural celebrations have to do with my modern, daily life?

As drawn as I was at first to the sabbats and the concept of celebrating nature, I went through that same ebb-and-flow and lack of personal, intimate connection. It took me many years to get in touch with the power of the sabbats in my own way, which has taken on the form of self-care, like much of my witchcraft practice. Now, my sabbat rituals are a time to check in and see how I've grown, what I've manifested in my life, and how I'm feeling since the last seasonal marker. It has been a natural evolution as I've developed daily spiritual practices that truly resonate with me and feel supportive.

I am a cottage witch, meaning I practice a holistic form of witchcraft that encompasses elements of the kitchen and garden with a focus on creating a sense of sanctuary. I'm a naturally high-energy person, often jumping from project to project with a difficult time turning off. Once I eventually came to understand this need for sanctuary that I have, both my spiritual path and the types of self-care that feel really nourishing all fell into place.

Understanding my needs has been and continues to be a process of trial and error, and in many ways, this book is composed of all the lessons I've learned (so far) along the way. (I say so far because the spiritual journey is not one with a destination!)

When I first began practicing, I did what all newbie witches do: I dove deep into the rabbit hole of the Internet and the relatively few published books on witchcraft that existed at the time and began researching. I wanted to know all about how to be a witch, how to practice spells and rituals, how to create a fancy grimoire, and how to follow the cycles of the moon in my life. It took me many years of practicing on and off to learn that the most valuable and supportive elements of my spirituality have little to do with what my practice looks like and far more to do with how it fulfills me.

The same goes for your self-care practice. There really are few distinctions between your spiritual and self-care practices. When you are exploring alternative spiritual paths like that of the witch, you are setting out on a journey to create your spirituality. When you are exploring the idea of incorporating greater self-care into your life, you are setting out on a journey to create the care that you need. There is no set path you must walk, no set practices you must do, and no set rules you must follow.

That can be exciting and liberating, but the weight of that many options can also be crushing. Witches have long been outcasts because they don't abide by the rules of society. This goes for both "real" witches and those accused of being witches by the church or state, like those executed in the witch trials of Salem and throughout Europe. In the twenty-first century, we have reclaimed what it means to be a witch, turned this once-negative word into one of empowerment and, yes, of self-care. We have taken on the mantle of outcast to honor the women who came before us, who chose to break the rules and create their own, when it was *not* the easiest or even safest lifestyle. It is often easier to follow someone else's rules, even if they don't feel quite right, than it is to do the hard work of creating the life and practices that actually make sense for you.

Witchcraft helps you to alchemize the status quo of self-care into a practice that is truly, deeply unique to you. A practice that honors your own individual needs and allows you to make up the rules as you see fit.

What does witchcraft have to do with self-care? Everything. Both are the journey toward fulfillment from *within*, instead of seeking answers from without.

WHO IS THE MODERN WITCH?

You might be wondering if this path is actually right for you. Are you a modern witch?

My short answer would be: probably.

To me, a modern witch is someone who knows she has the power to create her own reality. A woman who knows she is filled with the power of a goddess, a high priestess, and, most importantly, her own intuition.

A modern witch is someone who trusts herself implicitly—or is learning to—because we have all been conditioned by society and life to believe that our intuition is a faulty guidance system and that we need advice from outside of ourselves, especially from the established social leaders (conveniently). Most importantly, a modern witch is someone who declares themselves to be. This is the

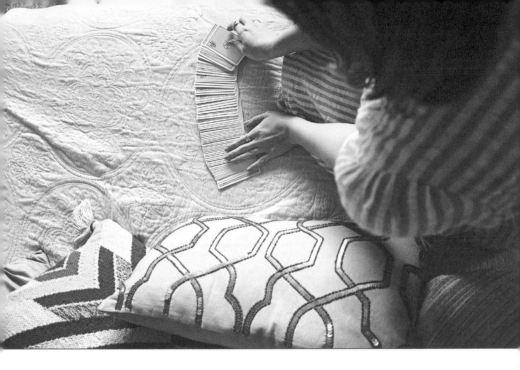

paramount way to know if you are a witch: if you feel that you are and you declare it to be so, whether privately to yourself or from the rooftops to the entire world, then you are a witch. There are no set beliefs a modern witch must hold and no set tools a modern witch must use. That is the beauty of witchcraft: the only path that truly exists is the one that is right for you.

You might have a picture in your head of what a witch is supposed to look like: perhaps a mysterious old woman who lives in a cottage in the woods and stirs her cauldron of herbs, brewing potions for mystical purposes. Maybe that's an image you aspire to or one that feels unattainable in your modern life. Maybe it's one that turns you off because it's constructed from a fairy tale instead of reality. Or maybe the picture in your head is one of a green-skinned, wart-nosed crone with a bad attitude and you're wondering why you would ever want to identify with her. Or maybe that crone fires you up and makes you want to be her, because you see the beauty in her wisdom and experience!

By contrast to these pop culture images, the modern witches that I know come in all varieties: a mystic goddess who lives part-time on a boat; a city-dwelling herbalist; a succulent-loving graphic designer; a mom with a successful business who expresses magick through her excellent fashion sense; an astrologer with a cat and a tiny apartment that's as magickal as she is. Some of these people call themselves witches, some do not, but all have the spirit of the modern witch. Their lifestyles and spiritual practices reflect their own personalities, their own interests and beliefs, the cities in which they live, and their varying needs for rest, community, trust in themselves, and connection to nature. If you were to ask each of them how self-care supports their path as a witch, I think you would get completely different and yet beautifully synchronistic answers.

In this way, we are all modern witches.

So, if you are wondering if this is the right path for you, my best advice is to try it. A sense of play is such an important part of self-care—the ability to play with ideas and use the imaginative ability that we lose at some point between childhood and adulting—so just allow yourself to play with your spiritual path. Spirituality has its deep and enlightening moments but there are also moments of play, moments of laughter, and moments of connection. A truly fulfilling path is relevant at every part of our lives—the serious moments, the absurd moments, the heartbreaking moments, and the raw, joyful moments, as well.

Creating your spiritual path, choosing to pursue the path that is truly fulfilling rather than what seems easiest, is an act of self-care. Therefore, the act of declaring yourself a witch is an act of self-care in and of itself. That's not because it's easy but rather *because* it's hard.

Being a witch is never going to be the easiest spiritual path. It can be tough to explain to other people what it is you believe and why you believe it, in a way that they can understand. You may face lectures from well-meaning but misguided people who believe you're on a path of evil temptation (a perspective they usually project from their own spirituality without stopping to try and understand yours).

It's also not easy to make up the rules. Like I said before, it seems liberating at first, but having to create your own belief system from the ground up can be quite daunting. There have to be some boundaries, even if they only make sense to you; without any rules, it becomes all too easy to fall off the spiritual bandwagon and stop practicing altogether (I've been there myself), because there is nothing to guide you back to your path when you stray. So, although there are no rules you *must* follow, you still have to find the boundaries of your own path and that takes a certain amount of dedication.

I don't say all this to discourage you from following the path of a witch or another alternative spirituality. Rather, I mention it to reinforce the fact that although it is often not an easy path to walk, it is one that can ultimately be far more fulfilling than following the rules and beliefs laid out by others. When you've put in the effort and dedicated yourself to creating a practice that actually fulfills you on a soul level, the rewards are unimaginable.

This is why witchcraft is a form of self-care and why integrating magickal rituals into your self-care practice can be so powerful. By making magick part of your self-care experience, you are heeding

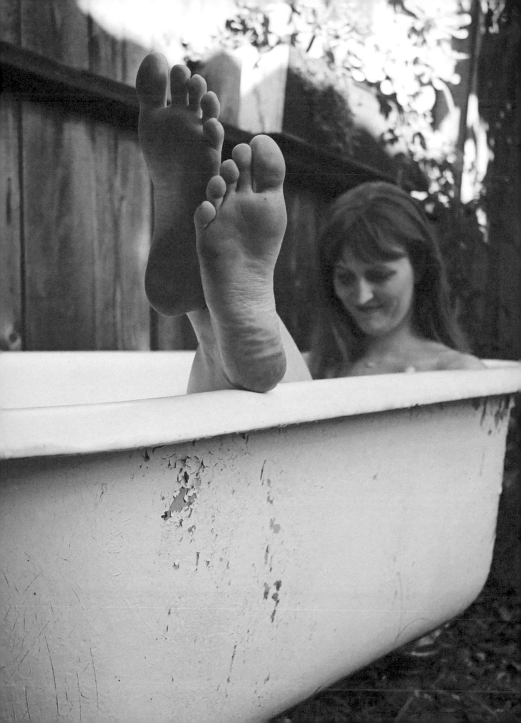

the call for something that feeds your soul on a deeper level than the pampering bubble baths and tea blends of your Pinterest feed. (Although, don't get me wrong, bubble baths, tea blends, and even Pinterest can be powerful magick themselves—all things we will talk about later in the book!)

This book is really a handbook, designed to give you the practical tools and techniques you will need to start crafting your own magickal self-care rituals. Sharing this kind of practical wisdom that gives you the tools to create rather than setting out rules and regulations to follow is my own personal mission. You'll learn about your self-care style through astrology in Chapter 3 on page 47; my own personal astrology shows me that my natural gifts are to share passion and individuality with the world—and to help others find their own. Although you will find some suggested rituals and recommendations for how to combine different practices, you will also find that this book is continually inviting you to think critically about your own path and beliefs and to apply the suggestions in a way that makes sense for you.

Everything in this book is adaptable and I encourage you to do just that. I recommend you start what is called a witch's grimoire, a book dedicated to your magickal practice, for your self-care journey, as you'll find lots of journal prompts and exercises to complete in this book. In this sacred text, your self-care grimoire, you can record answers to all the questions in this book, as well as define your rituals over time. Though it is a sacred book of magick and witchcraft, you can use anything for your grimoire that feels right to you; don't be afraid to use a notebook, a three-ring binder, or even to keep your grimoire digitally. I recommend not thinking too hard about it as many people get hung up on what their grimoire should be, instead of how to use it.

There are dozens of factors that affect what kind of self-care you need in your life, and that will definitely evolve over time. Here are just a few of the things that may affect your self-care needs:

- Your mental and physical health
- Your emotional state at any given time
- Your lifestyle, including how much time you have to practice and how much space and privacy you have to practice in
- Your spiritual and religious beliefs
- Your personal astrology

The combination of these factors makes you who you are: we are the sum of many, many parts of ourselves. Your health and emotions impact your ability to do pretty much anything in your life, whether for yourself or others. Being consciously aware of that impact and learning to live in flow with your physical, mental, and emotional rhythms is a powerful way to step into your fullest potential.

Your lifestyle has likely evolved much over the years: you probably live very differently than you did when you were a child or when you were in college and you will live differently when you have children or live with a partner. Whatever stage of life you are in now, you've probably had earlier stages when your lifestyle looked quite different than it does at this point, and you will likely have more mature stages in the future. The space you live in, the people and animals you live with, your schedule and that of those around you—all of these factors have a massive impact on your spiritual and self-care needs.

Your beliefs are so important, too! People often think that our beliefs don't change over time but that's patently untrue. The experiences we have throughout our lives shape what we believe. People change political parties and religions all the time and there's a reason. Some great catalyst in their lives has shown them that they were on the wrong path for them (not necessarily the wrong path for anyone else, but the wrong path for *them*).

And then there is your cosmic makeup. Your personal astrology, the map to your highest potential that the universe laid out at the moment of your birth: your astrological natal chart. The unique placement of planets and asteroids in your chart is the source of great insight into who you are at your core. Your cosmic makeup does not dictate who you are. Rather, it shows you who you always knew you could be, and more importantly, gives you the tools to reach the potential inside of you.

BELIEFS

Witchcraft is a spiritual path and although we're not talking so much in this book about *religious* faith, even the most alternative spiritual path reflects a set of beliefs.

Your beliefs might include faith in a god or deity, or they might not.

Your beliefs might include faith in spirits, ancestors or faeries, or they might not.

For the purposes of this book, it doesn't really matter what your beliefs are. What does matter is that you're continually getting curious about what it is you believe in that moment and you can turn to those beliefs in not only difficult times but joyful ones, too. Your beliefs affect your self-care practice in that they are going to inform what it is you find fulfilling. For example, if you believe that food is the root of all love and nourishment, then focusing on your own nutrition and being sure others are fed and healthy might be what is most fulfilling for you. Cooking food for your own family or volunteering time at a shelter or food bank might fulfill those needs. But if you believe that love comes from the divine and that we need to have a relationship with your god/goddess in order to become enlightened in this life, then prayer and pilgrimage might be what fulfills that deep well of longing within you.

Your beliefs are the set of boundaries, faith, and tools that you've set out for yourself as you pursue your spiritual path. Hopefully, those beliefs were crafted by getting to know what your own spiritual needs are and choosing the tools to meet those needs. Sometimes, though, we create a spiritual system in our lives not out of what we need but out of what we think. You might think *yes, I should pray to a deity*, or *yes, I should practice meditation*, but do you stop to ask yourself: why? Why do you feel called to do this, and is it inspired by the source of your needs or by the influence of an outside entity? (It can be both, for the record.)

Ask yourself these questions to explore the ways that your spiritual path is fulfilling your needs (or not):

How did you discover the spiritual path you are currently on? What led you here?

_____

_____

_____

What are your mental and emotional needs? What makes you feel nourished mentally and emotionally?

_____

_____

_____

In what ways do you feel that you benefit from support from a higher power (whether that's a deity, spirit, ancestor, your higher self, etc.)?

_____

_____

_____

Why do you seek a spiritual path? What support or enlightenment does your spiritual path provide you with?

_____

_____

_____

Make a list of all your spiritual beliefs that you can think of. Write down any deities or entities that you believe in, the tools you like to use in your spiritual practice and why, the feelings that you get when you practice a ritual or spell—all of it.

_____

_____

_____

_____

_____

_____

_____

_____

_____

Now, compare the list you've made to the answers you gave to each of the questions above. Do you have any needs that are not being fulfilled by your current spiritual practice? Are you practicing any elements that aren't really fulfilling any particular needs?

_____

_____

_____

_____

_____

Asking yourself these questions is going to open up the why and the how and the deep roots of your spirituality. Once you know what your needs are, creating your spiritual practice becomes a process of filling in the blanks. This is truly what witchcraft has to do with self-care, for witchcraft is the practice of creating and transforming your reality, and self-care is the tool (the wand, if you will) with which you transform yourself from the inside out.

MENTAL, PHYSICAL & EMOTIONAL HEALTH

Of the many factors that can affect your self-care needs, your health, in all its various facets, is one of the biggest. At its most basic level, self-care literally refers to your health and to taking care of your mind and body. This term actually originated from a movement to care for ourselves *before* we need medical attention instead of seeking medical treatment for symptoms as the primary form of health care.

We all need certain support to keep our minds and bodies functioning at their optimal capacity. Everything from stress levels to hormone imbalances to dietary sensitivities can impact the way we function both mentally and physically, and all of these ailments are becoming increasingly more common in our world. This will apply especially if you have particular health concerns, but caring for your mind and body is important even if you consider yourself to be perfectly healthy.

In this way, seemingly mundane acts like visiting a therapist and keeping up with diet and exercise routines can be a major part of your self-care practice, regardless of the spiritual activities we'll be discussing in this book. There's nothing that says these "mundane" acts of self-care can't be spiritual, too, though! In fact, any activity that supports, nourishes, and fulfills you can be a form of spiritual self-care. For example, eating a healthy, seasonal diet that nourishes your unique dietary needs could tie into your celebrations of the sabbats by preparing holiday meals with plants that are in season and which nourish your body and spirit.

I also think it's important to talk about the fact that we all have unique physical needs. For example, I'm allergic to chamomile. It makes me sneeze like crazy! Know what every self-care book seems to recommend? A cup of chamomile tea before bed to help you relax and fall asleep more easily. Well, that's just a no-go for me, as are chamomile candles and essential oils. That doesn't mean I'm doomed to a life of insomnia and restless sleep, just that herbs like lavender or valerian are going to be better choices for me.

Especially if you are allergic to a common ingredient like I am or if you have another unique dietary or health restriction, just know that you can always adapt suggested self-care practices to your own needs. Just because your needs are different than that of the masses does not mean you can't create beautiful and nourishing self-care rituals for yourself!

A truly supportive self-care practice will fulfill complex combinations of mental, physical, emotional, and spiritual needs. Take a step back and think about your health objectively. So often, we, especially women, experience daily discomforts that we dismiss as part of "being a woman" or "getting older" or we just blame it on bad takeout and move on with our lives. But our optimal health is so much more complex than we give it credit for and operating at your healthiest self may be a level of vibrancy you didn't even know you could experience.

Answer the following questions in your journal and take the time to really think about how you feel on a day-to-day basis:

Do you consider yourself to be "healthy"? Why or why not?

_____

_____

_____

Are there health concerns that have arisen in your life? How did you handle them? Are they currently under control or have you not had a chance to address them directly?

_____

_____

_____

What mental and emotional triggers come up for you? How do you react to them? Do you currently have a plan in place for how to handle unexpectedly triggering situations? What can you do to prepare yourself to handle those situations?

_____

_____

_____

What seemingly minor discomforts do you experience regularly?

_____

_____

_____

LIFESTYLE

Your lifestyle also has a huge impact on the needs you have to fulfill within yourself. A lot of times we think of spiritual self-care as somewhat static, something that serves our most fundamental needs. It's true that who we are at our most fundamental core doesn't really change throughout our lives, though we may evolve and grow into stronger versions of ourselves. But our environments are always changing and the way you live your life should be at the heart of your ever-changing self-care practice.

Lifestyle encompasses everything from career to living situation to relationships to finances. Let's discuss these one at a time.

Your career, or at least what you spend your days doing, even if that's volunteerism or educating yourself, likely takes up the bulk of your time. In the US, we typically spend more time during the day with our coworkers than with our own families (sad, but true). Your self-care needs can be affected by the hours you work, your physical working environment, your relationships with your colleagues, and how much you do or do not enjoy the work you're doing.

Long or late hours, an unhealthy or dangerous working environ-ment, bitter coworker relationships, and disliking your job can all lead to great dissatisfaction (obviously). In situations like that, your self-care practice is going to need to really step up and fill in the gaps created by your unfulfilling career. Maybe your self-care practice needs to include looking for ways to create a different situation for yourself, but don't neglect your actual self-care in the meantime. Even if you're working to get out of a bad situation, taking the time to care for yourself will go a long way in giving you the energy to move forward.

Your home space is another big factor. Your living environment has a huge impact on how happy, healthy, and connected you are likely to feel. This includes the physical amount of space you have to call your own, the things within that space, the people and animals you share that space with, and the level of safety and comfort you feel there.

Having a sacred space to practice your spirituality can be a really supportive element of self-care, but it's not always possible. Maybe your space is just too small for an altar, or maybe you share it with

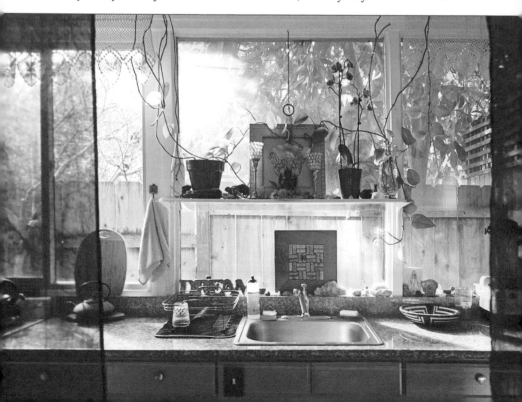

people who are not supportive of your path. Clutter, bad smells, and unfinished chores can all make you feel trapped and unable to relax in your space. Taking care of the most mundane of chores, like washing and putting away the clothes or dishes or vacuuming the floor, can be an act of self-care, as it frees you up to focus on more important things. Creating a home self-care practice is also about finding room for the sacred in your existing physical surroundings, even if it's not your perfect, ideal vision of what that is "supposed" to look like.

Relationships are perhaps one of the biggest factors in how your lifestyle affects your self-care needs, including romantic relationships, friendships, and family relationships and just how you relate to other people in general. The people who you surround yourself with greatly impact your attitude, habits, and even beliefs. Positive, supportive relationships lift you up, help you to see your greatest potential, and open you up to unlimited possibilities. Negative relationships can really drag you down, though, and keep you in cycles of limiting beliefs about yourself and your potential.

Your self-care practice needs to address the ways in which you relate to others, how you take on their needs and attitudes, and what you need to do to protect yourself while remaining open. It's important to remember that even the most supportive relationships can have their pitfalls and that sometimes you may just need space and solitude. If that's you, then taking the alone time that you need should be a major part of your self-care practice.

Of all the factors that can affect your self-care needs, finances is perhaps the most mundane and yet it has some of the greatest potential to afflict you with stress and worry. Debt, loans, and just paying the monthly bills can be a huge source of stress because it always trickles down and affects something else; maybe your dream career just isn't paying enough or doesn't provide benefits; maybe your rent or mortgage is becoming unaffordable; or the stress of debt is beginning to take a toll on your relationships. Your self-care practice needs to address any source of stress that's coming into your life and disrupting your potential for harmonious manifestation of the life you want, and finances can be a big part of that stress.

Take a bird's-eye view of your life and see if you can look at each of these areas individually. Ask yourself the following questions:

Does your current work or career feel fulfilling? Why or why not? What would change if your daily work fulfilled your needs for creative expression, helping others, or some other desire?

_____

_____

_____

Does your current home space feel nourishing? Do you have a sacred space to practice your spirituality? Do you worry about needing to hide your spirituality at home?

_____

_____

_____

Do your current relationships feel positive and uplifting? Why or why not? How can you intentionally adapt the way you relate to others to be more supportive of your own needs?

_____

_____

_____

Does your current financial situation feel safe and supportive? Why or why not? What practical actions can you take to alleviate financial strain if you are feeling it?

_____

_____

_____

WHO YOU ARE AT YOUR CORE

Your spiritual and self-care needs are also affected by simply who you are at your core. Your habits, the way you communicate, the way you receive intuitive information, your unique brand of play and creativity—all of these things combine to make up what makes you uniquely you. Journaling prompts like those in this chapter can be a magickal way to start better understanding who you are, as is taking a close look at your astrological natal chart, which we'll be doing in Chapter 3 on page 47.

However, the most powerful tool you have at your disposal is your own intuition. When you ask yourself a question such as _what are my most fundamental needs?_ and all of the other questions in this chapter, you are asking it of your intuition. The answer you receive when you're really in flow, when you've allowed yourself to get out of your head and out of your own way? That answer is coming from your intuition.

Often, you may be surprised by the answers you receive from your intuition. They don't always make sense on the surface but when you dig down deeper, you'll always find that there are layers of yourself you haven't met yet. Aspects of yourself you haven't explored, that your intuition will be delighted to give you a tour of, now that you're ready and listening. Your intuition is always there and it's just a matter of tuning into it and really beginning to pay attention.

When you take the time to tune into your intuitive downloads and to really process the information you receive, you're getting deep with *yourself*. You're doing the shadow work of setting aside your expectations and the expectations of others and allowing your intuition to show you what you *really* need. What is *really* right for you.

> **What is shadow work, you might be wondering?** *Shadows are the Jungian concept of the parts of ourselves that we may not even be conscious of or that we actively dislike. These are often judgments we pass against others, even though we see the same "flaw" in ourselves, or attitudes that we have without even realizing it. Shadow work is the process of learning to understand these aspects of ourselves and either release or learn to live harmoniously with them.*

Again, what's right for you is not necessarily right for anyone else. Understanding this distinction is so, so important. Your intuition is not governed by anyone else's sense of right and wrong or good and bad—it is led only by your own sense of those concepts. This is why we're starting off in the next chapter with getting in touch with your intuition and learning to trust yourself, so that you can discover what magickal self-care practices are truly going to resonate with you!

To bring this all back around, let's ask again, what does witchcraft have to do with self-care? At its core, witchcraft is the *craft* of connection.

Connecting with and caring for nature.

Connecting with and caring for animals.

Connecting with and caring for our ancestors and spirit guides.

Connecting with and caring for the people we love.

Connecting with and caring for perfect strangers who also deserve our respect.

It is the path of coming to understand the connections between all living things and the spiritual force that binds us together. And even if that concept resonates on a soul level, most of us have abandoned the act of connecting with and caring for *ourselves*. It is so easy to allow all of your obligations to consume you and your time, and to give over a part of yourself in the process.

Witchcraft and self-care are two parallel paths of reclaiming who you are, reclaiming the awareness of what you need, and, most importantly, reclaiming the wisdom of how to fulfill your own needs so that you can live in flow and step into your fullest potential.

Chapter 2
FIND WHAT RESONATES WITH YOU

The very first step in creating any ritual is to find what resonates with you. This is what we are going to spend most of this book doing, playing with different ideas and tools and experimenting with how they make you feel. After all, just as a predetermined spiritual path is unlikely to be as fulfilling as one of your own making, self-care rituals are not one-size-fits-all.

I like to think of self-care as falling into two very broad categories: internal and external. You can think of this as the care of your inner self through nourishment of your mental and emotional health and the care of your outer self through nourishment of your physical body, but it's more than that. We also require self-care that comes from within, the kind of care that involves self-reflection and awareness, as well as self-care that comes from outside of ourselves, from the natural world or the divine.

Breaking these internal and external categories down a bit further, internal self-care encompasses the mind, body, and intuition while external self-care encompasses connections to nature and expressions of devotion.

External self-care may sound like a contradiction. If it's called *self-care*, doesn't that inherently mean that it can only come from within? There's a bit of an oxymoron here but it's true: self-care comes from many sources. It is our awareness of our need for various forms of external nourishment that makes those things part of a self-care practice. So, for example, if going for a hike or visiting a temple feels really nourishing for you, your awareness that you need to be sure to regularly schedule time to do those things is how you incorporate them into your self-care rituals.

Let's look at each of these areas of self-care, which we'll explore in greater depth later in this book.

INTERNAL SELF-CARE: MIND, BODY & INTUITION

Self-care that nurtures your mind and body are perhaps the most "traditional" forms of self-care, if there is such a thing. Self-care as a term has a lot of political and feminist associations, so it hasn't been in existence as it is in our current collective consciousness for very long. Its original iteration was that of caring for ourselves when our broken, patriarchal medical system could not and therefore referred to our mental and physical health.

There are countless examples of how women's health is not taken seriously by the medical establishment. Common women's health issues like endometriosis and Hashimoto's can take an average of five years and multiple doctors to diagnose, because the symptoms are often dismissed as a "normal" part of the menstrual cycle or a mysterious hormonal imbalance. This is partly because medical doctors often notoriously dismiss the complaints of their female patients and partly because the research just hasn't been done: we don't have all the information we need to be able to easily and painlessly diagnose many of these disorders. Even when they are diagnosable, there are often few, invasive, or ineffective treatments.

I experienced this fairly recently when I broke out in some kind of terrible, reactionary rash. I was never diagnosed with anything but it took five separate doctors (each with their own theory as to what was wrong with me), an emergency room visit, and several painful shots and blood tests to finally at least treat my symptoms. I still don't know what caused the reaction in the first place; at the time, finding out wasn't anyone's priority. Most women I know have a story like this: an instance when they suffered and the system wasn't capable of supporting them. So, the idea of self-care came into play; if our doctors can't take care of us, let's take care of ourselves. We started to take up self-reflective journaling and paying attention to our nutrition, not just for the sake of our weight but for the sake of really feeling good, feeling powerful in our bodies.

Over time, though, "self-care" became trendy and started to look like pedicures and bubble baths. Businesses started to capitalize on the phrase and promote their products and cosmetics as the paraphernalia of self-care.

Honestly, I'm not against this. Bubble baths are great.

But it's important to understand where we started and what taking care of our minds and bodies really means. There is a physical aspect, definitely. In the next chapter, we'll be looking at your personal astrology to understand your self-care style and for some signs, caring for and pampering the physical body is a must. It's about so much more than pampering, though.

Caring for your physical body means both eating things that make you feel healthy and also eating things that make you feel indulgent and pampered. Caring for your physical body means both having great sex and setting boundaries around when and where you feel good being touched or not. Caring for your physical body means using cosmetic products that are aligned with your values (such as companies that use recycled packaging or do not practice animal testing), and that make you feel beautiful in your own eyes.

And what about your mind? Your mind is expansive and limitless and so is your care of it. Sure, mental self-care can mean journaling, self-reflection, and meditation and those are all things we're going to talk more about. But it can also mean practicing aromatherapy to calm yourself, listening to music or making music, or even picking up an adult coloring book (trendy does not equal bad)! Cutting unhealthy relationships out of your life and putting a stop to conversations that make you uncomfortable are forms of caring for your mind. Anything that puts your mind at ease and allows you to be truly relaxed in your own company is mental self-care.

Ask yourself these questions to dig deeper into what kinds of mental and physical self-care practices are right for you:

Where do you regularly experience pain or fatigue in your body? Do you have any injuries that you need to care for?

_____

_____

_____

Think really intentionally about your diet. What foods are you currently consuming that feel truly nourishing?

_____

_____

_____

Do you ever feel mentally exhausted? What brings that feeling on?

_____

_____

_____

What activities make you feel truly calm and at peace? How often do you do these?

_____

_____

_____

Your mind and body are the tools and the sacred spaces that you always have on hand. Even when you're apart from your most sacred altars and unable to practice your most treasured rituals, you always have yourself. Being able to tap into your body, ask yourself what you need, and then follow through in order to provide it, is the most powerful act of self-care you can give yourself. But finding that ability within yourself requires one more crucial ingredient: trusting your intuition.

Every aspect of your mental, spiritual, and physical experience can have an impact on the kinds of self-care you need. That's because self-care fills the various gaps that you have in your life, the spaces where you feel unfulfilled or unsupported, which change depending on your circumstances. A magickal self-care practice relies on trusting your intuition in knowing where those gaps in your life are and how they need to be addressed.

It can be easy to "get in your head" about self-care and think that you need to be doing certain things or that certain activities are supposed to make you feel a certain way. This is following your ego and your head, listening to outside sources about what your self-care should look like. The more supportive and sustainable way to create a self-care practice is by following your intuition and your heart. Your self-care practice doesn't have to make sense to anyone else; it's only purpose is to serve *your* needs.

The first step here is to get in touch with your intuition and then to start learning to really trust it. This will not be an overnight process, but rather an ongoing journey toward trust. Your intuition is always there; it's just a matter of paying it the attention it deserves. You do not have to be psychic or clairvoyant to get in touch with your intuition. Intuitive power is something that everyone has. It's the instinct that lets you know when someone isn't being truthful or authentic with you. It's that little voice in the back of your head that tells you when something is good or bad.

Now, it's not necessarily the little voice that tells you when something is *right* or *wrong*; that's your conscience, and your conscience is affected by many factors outside of yourself. Conscience is developed through social conditioning from the time we are small children. We are told which acts and words are wrong and which activities we are supposed to engage in if we are good people. Some of these are fairly innate and universal across most

BODY SCAN MEDITATION

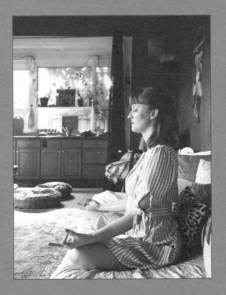

Body scan meditation can be a really great way to connect your mind and body and to become more aware of yourself and your needs.

Find a comfortable place to lay down and close your eyes. Place your hands in a natural place such as at your sides or folded on your belly. Take a deep, cleansing breath in through your nose and release it through your mouth.

Starting at the top of your head, begin to notice the sensation of being in a physical body. Scan your body from the crown of your head, slowly down your forehead. Bring awareness to and then relax every part of your body as you scan it. Relax your eyes, your tongue, your jaw. Relax your shoulders and arms, sinking more deeply into the ground.

Relax your chest, your body, your stomach, your hips. Relax your legs, allowing your knees to fall gently open if that's comfortable.

Scan all the way down to the tips of your toes, bringing awareness and then relaxation to every part of your body. As you scan, pay attention to the physical sensations you experience, where your body aches or feels stiff. So often, we arc not even aware of how we're feeling until we stop and really ask our bodies what they need!

cultures, such as theft or more severe acts like murder. But many of the things we are told are "wrong" are actually constructs of the religious and socio-political culture around us.

Your intuition is what tells you when your conscience is wrong. To use witchcraft itself as the example, your intuition is what may be telling you that the path of the modern witch is right for you even as your ego-driven conscience flares up and warns you that this path is untraditional, taboo, or that your friends or family might not respect it.

It's important to acknowledge your ego when this happens, not repress it, as it will only flare up more vigorously in other ways if ignored. By acknowledging and gently but firmly denying your ego when that's what is needed, you grant your intuition greater power in the process of making decisions and processing information.

But why is that important? What makes getting in touch with your intuition so powerful?

Intuition is the expression of your subconscious mind. Your subconscious knows far more than you do, as our brains are only capable of being aware of a small fraction of the information that we take in every day. Estimates range in the millions to billions of pieces of information that we process every second, but we are only aware of a few thousand. That means that your brain takes in literally billions of bits of information every day that you may retain without an explicit awareness of them.

In this way, intuition is the expression of the information that resides in your subconscious as you begin to become aware of something that you already know. Intuition is also thought of as the voice of your higher self. Your higher self is the version of you that is in alignment with your highest potential. It's important to realize that potential is not just your ideal career path or the version of your life in which you are the most "successful." Your higher self is also in alignment with your potential for creativity, joy, love, and self-awareness.

In order to receive guidance from your higher self toward manifesting your highest potential, you are going to need to get in touch with your intuition. That little voice that tells you when you're on the right path is how your higher self communicates with you. When you are in tune with your intuition, you'll receive information through these channels; we call them intuitive hits, downloads, or nudges but the way that you receive information from your intuition and your higher self will be entirely unique to you.

Your intuition can guide you in every aspect of your life and it is definitely an important element of developing your magickal self-care practice. Though we will be looking at astrology, your personal interests, and other ways to find what acts of self-care resonate with you, your intuition is the most important tool in your kit. Only your intuition can tell you if something feels right, if it feels supportive and nourishes your soul.

Even if every sign in the world seems to point to one thing as the ultimate way to express love for yourself, if your intuition says "no" then you need to be able to trust that. Sometimes, trusting your intuition can be scary. Sometimes, your intuition tells you to do something that seems ridiculous or silly or even foolish. A truly supportive self-care practice is about honoring your own needs, no matter how ridiculous, silly, or foolish they might seem to an outsider. Only you and your higher self know the truth of what is supportive for you.

That's why getting in touch with your intuition is so important. I can give you all the tools and techniques for creating a self-care practice, for expressing devotion to self-love, and for discovering your inner witch, but if you're acting out of sync with your intuition and your higher self, those tools will only lead you down a path of disappointment. As we progress toward creating your own magickal self-care practice, I want you to check every possibility against your own intuitive power. Ask yourself if each tool, each ritual, and each technique would be a supportive part of self-care for you.

That's not to say that the roles you play in your life are not a part of you or that your relationships are insignificant; rather, your inner witch is the person you are when you're alone. We all have aspects of ourselves we keep hidden even from those we are closest to. Your evening ritual should feel nourishing to the person you are when you're alone with your thoughts.

Don't take my word for it: always ask your higher self!

In the next pages, we will explore a few different rituals you can use to connect with your intuition. These rituals are extremely adaptable to your own practice and beliefs and can be used interchangeably. I recommend that you try them all out and see what works for you—you won't know what helps you get in touch with your inner wisdom until you try!

DREAM JOURNALING

My personal favorite suggestion to start your intuitive journey is through dream journaling. This simple yet powerful technique is a great way to start training your brain and your ego that your intuition is important enough to pay attention to.

Choose a notebook to use for your dream journaling. On the first night of your practice, dedicate the journal to your purpose with the following ritual. This ritual will be most powerful on the night of the new moon, as new moons are a great time for starting new things and dedicating yourself to new intentions, but you can perform it at any time.

Light three black candles, as black is the color of the new moon, the time when we set intentions.

Don't have three candles? Just light one. Don't have black candles? Use white. Don't have any candles? Try battery-operated or visualize a white light surrounding the journal instead! Everything about the rituals suggested in this book is adaptable to your reality.

Place your hands on the journal and close your eyes. Focus on your intention of getting in touch with your intuition so that you can understand yourself better. When you are ready, open your eyes and turn to the first page of the journal.

Write a dedication on the first page such as "I dedicate this journal to the purpose of connecting with my intuition" or "I dedicate this grimoire to pursuing my intuitive power." Your dedication should really come from the heart and feel natural. You could also decorate this page or draw a sigil (a symbol), of intuition.

Place the journal beside your bed.

Place an amethyst crystal on top of the journal, as amethyst is the crystal of dreams and intuition, and have a pen readily available.

When you wake up in the morning, reach for the journal first thing. It's important that you write your dreams down right away, as we start to forget our dreams very quickly once we wake. Be sure not to reach for your phone or any other distractions before writing down your dreams. Record all of the details that you remember.

Now, take a moment for reflection. Why do you think you had this dream? Was there something in your day or week before that may have inspired it? Was it a nightmare or a dream you've had before? I suggest doing this reflection entirely intuitively; although sometimes classic symbols appear in our dreams, this practice is about getting in touch with your own intuition so it's important to trust that you can understand the deeper meaning of your dreams on your own without referring to a dream dictionary.

Do this practice of recording your dreams and reflecting on them every morning, as often as you can. On mornings when you simply don't remember your dreams at all, write down "No dream recollection" or simply "I don't remember." This trains your brain that this information is worth remembering. If it happens frequently, try not to get frustrated. Your intuition may just need to be accessed in a different way.

ITEMS FOR YOUR NIGHTSTAND DREAM ALTAR

Creating an altar on your nightstand is a powerful way to remind yourself to connect with your intuition in even mundane moments like preparing for bed. This reminder again starts to train your brain that this intention is worthy of your time. You can include any items on your dream altar that speak to you intuitively, but here are a few suggestions:

- Lavender for sleep and relaxation (bundles of fresh lavender, sachets of dried lavender, or lavender essential oil in a diffuser or roller ball)

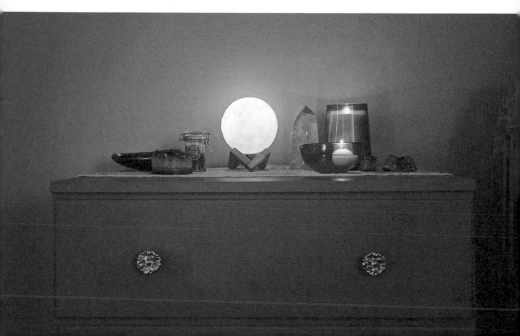

- Mugwort for intuitive dreams (a sachet of dried mugwort or mugwort incense)
- Amethyst for dreams and intuition (raw chunks of amethyst, polished stones, or massage wands)
- Candles scented with relaxing scents like lavender—just be sure to always blow out the candles before falling asleep!
- Representations of the moon, which rules over dreams and intuition, such as a moon lamp or a picture or drawing of the moon
- Representations of the element of water, which rules intuition, such as a bowl of water with a floating candle, a seashell, even a glass of lemon water to drink in the morning (as lemons are ruled by the moon as well)

DAILY DIVINATION

If dream journaling is not resonating with you, a daily divination practice is another great way to get in touch with your intuition. Divination is the practice of utilizing an established tool to divine the knowledge you are seeking. Some people use divination to attempt to tell the future, but the modern understanding of these tools is that they are best used to help us understand what our intuition is trying to tell us.

A few examples of divinatory tools include:

- Tarot cards
- Oracle cards
- Runes
- Pendulums

- Crystal balls or gazing mirrors
- Tasseography (reading tea leaves)

You can use any of these tools on a daily basis. Typically, when you use a divination tool, you ask a question that you are seeking the answer to. For example, you might be asking about how to find your ideal romantic partner or whether it would serve you to take a new job. When you use these tools daily though, not only do you come to understand your intuitive nudges better about those larger questions, you can also ask smaller, more general questions to guide your day.

I recommend simply asking yourself *what do I need to know for today?* and then consulting your favorite divination tool to guide you. It's important to remember that this is intuitive—a guidebook from your tarot deck or symbol dictionary may help you understand the broader message of the tools but you want to trust your intuition first. I usually like to freewrite a paragraph or two about what I think the message of the tool is for that day.

If you are engaging in a dream journaling practice, you can write down your dream reflection and divination reflection on the same page and start to find patterns and correlations between the two.

EXTERNAL SELF-CARE: NATURE & DEVOTION

I love to do surveys of the women I connect with on social media and on my website www.witchoflupinehollow.com to get their feedback and learn more about their perspective on magick, witchcraft, self-care, and other topics. In one such survey, I asked these women what it means to live a magickal life, in their own words. About 25 percent of those who responded to this particular survey said having a magickal life means having some kind of connection to nature. It wasn't a surprising result, really, as one of the most common questions I receive is about how to connect with nature when you live in an urban area or don't have access to the wilderness.

There is even a witchcraft path called that of the "wild witch," a person who explores their connection not just to herbs and the garden and the tamed versions of nature, but to the wild, unrestrained natural world which is often harder for our society to accept. We, as a culture, have spent literally hundreds of generations learning to tame the wilderness.

Our hunter-gatherer ancestors tamed wild beasts and settled in villages for the first time around ten thousand years ago. Myths arose around the dangers of lurking in the forests and the fear around what lay outside the village walls only grew over the millennia. By the Middle Ages and the Renaissance, a deep-seated distrust of all things wild had taken root within western culture.

Witches are associated with that same wildness that was so feared (and still is). Those accused of witchcraft during the witch trials of the sixteenth and seventeenth centuries often lived on the outskirts of town or were outcasts in some way. Women who lived alone were certainly considered suspicious, as were those who practiced healing with herbs and plants. Many people relied on those healers, as physicians were few and far between and often woefully inadequate. But even as they relied on these healers and midwives to heal them and treat their ailments, people often turned on them as soon as it was felt they had misused their power, or if the milk went "mysteriously" sour from being left out too long (and surely someone needed to be blamed and hanged for it).

The average person in the sixteenth century didn't understand how healers could take common herbs and plants growing in their own garden and mash them up into pastes, ointments, tonics, and tinctures to heal their diseases, and so those same healers became targets for abuse and persecution. Honestly, not that much has changed (although thankfully we don't hang herbalists anymore), but in the twenty-first century, our cultural knowledge of nature has waned far more than it had even during the time of the witch trials, to our detriment.

Returning to the idea of self-care as a counterpoint to the patriarchal health-care system, a knowledge of how herbs and oils can heal us or prevent us from becoming sick in the first place is powerful stuff. Learning to do the work of harvesting, drying, chopping, boiling, and speaking and praying over the herbs that have the power to heal us is a way of connecting with the wildness that predates our fear-based society. It's also a way of connecting with the women who were burned and hanged in earlier centuries for this same knowledge and of reclaiming their power.

It's about more than just the physical ways which the natural world can affect our bodies, however. Self-care through nature is also about healing ourselves of the twenty-first-century information pollution that invades our space on a constant basis. Believe it or not, I'm not actually of the mind that we are too inundated by various kinds of media; I think our ability to connect with people on the other side of the world, on all sides of the political and spiritual spectrum, and with all kinds of interests and needs is insanely powerful and, really, quite beautiful. We shouldn't be spending all our time lamenting the "good old days" back when we could more easily remain ignorant of what was happening in the world around us, but since we do live in a world of constant media and of updates on world news and politics which are often, frankly, depressing, it's more important than ever to disconnect mindfully. I have definitely been guilty of shutting out all news because it's too upsetting, confusing, or seems irrelevant to my existence. I know so many people who have shut down their social media accounts, for a variety of reasons. In some ways, shutting it all out can be a form of self-care in and of itself, but if you do this without intention, you're cutting yourself off from some of the most powerful forms of connection that exist in our modern world. The most powerful ways of connecting with each other that have *ever* existed.

This is where nature comes in: spending time in nature (or connecting with nature in a way that makes sense for your lifestyle) is probably the single most powerful way to mindfully disconnect from our modern reality. Then you can return, invigorated, and ready to reconnect in meaningful ways.

Like I said, one of the most common questions I receive from modern witches is about how to connect with nature when they don't, for example, live in a cottage in the forest with a thatched roof and a magical talking cat. This is a common, and understandable, misconception. Connecting with nature doesn't have to mean spending hours wandering through the forest, tracking small animals, picking berries, and identifying every plant you find along your path (although that sounds like a magickal way to spend an afternoon).

Rather, connecting with nature can mean sipping a cup of herbal tea or diffusing essential oils. It can mean going for a hike in a national park, but it can also mean going for a walk along the paved

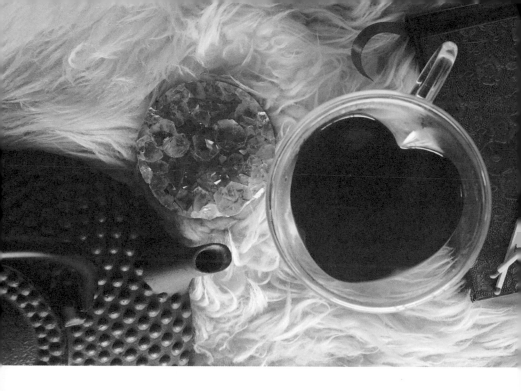

path through your local dog park. It can mean noticing the seasonal changes reflected in the changing colors of the trees along your commute. It can even show up in indoor activities: taking an herbal foot bath or facial steam, tending to potted plants, or cooking with fresh herbs and spices.

Connecting with nature and unleashing your inner wild woman can become an integral part of your daily life, likely without too many significant changes to your lifestyle. It's about noticing nature, respecting nature, and being a part of nature.

As you consider how you feel drawn to nature, ask yourself these questions:

What kind of natural space feels most relaxing for you, (e.g., a wild English garden or manicured French garden, a forest, a beach, etc.)?

_____

_____

_____

Is there anywhere you've ever visited that as soon as you entered the space, you felt immediately at peace?

_____

_____

_____

How do you engage with nature (including through plants, herbs, and oils) on a regular basis?

_____

_____

_____

Devotion is the act of expressing love and dedication to a person, thing, idea, or deity. Often, we think of devotion in terms of romantic love or worship of a god. In those contexts, devotion is the way we express our love for and faith in the person we love or the god we worship. But you can be devoted to almost anything. Perhaps you are devoted to a certain political cause. Perhaps you are devoted to your family, whether your actual relatives or the friends you've chosen as your family. Perhaps you are devoted to good food, putting healthy meals on the table for yourself and loved ones. Or maybe your devotion is to educating yourself, honoring the cycles of nature, or paying homage to your ancestors.

When you stop and think about it, there are probably a handful of ideas which you are most devoted to and which you feel most called to honor and express in your life. Self-care is the act of making sure you have the opportunity to express that devotion. When asked what things they care about most in life, most people can answer with a few things pretty readily: their children or family, their work, their political beliefs, their art. But when asked how much time they spend on those things, most people quibble that they just don't have the space in their life, around career and cooking dinner and all the other little tasks that take up their day. But that's the thing: if you don't have time or space for the things that you care about most, what is the point of all the other things you fill your day with? That's why making sure that you carve out time in your day (or even your week or month) to express devotion to the things that you feel most deeply about is one of the ultimate forms of self care.

Devotion can be supportive and nourishing in a few different ways. It can offer you guidance and insight, through the power of prayer or meditation. It can offer you comfort, through worship of a higher power or communicating with loved ones. It can offer a sense of connection with something larger than yourself, a common thread amongst the collective. Devotion can also be an act of creativity, of expressing yourself in wild, joyful, and ecstatic ways, of fulfilling the higher purpose of your soul. For example, in my own spiritual practice, I express devotion through the power of the stars. Astrology and the moon cycle have long been a part of my path and this is the area I feel most connected with and attuned to. Even when I get out of the habit of pulling a daily oracle card or fall off the wagon with my tea rituals, I always seem to know what sign or phase the moon is in and what's happening in the sky. I often think of the world around me in terms of what signs rule the different aspects of life (like Leo ruling a sunny, joyful day).

My monthly new and full moon rituals are a checkpoint to see how I'm doing, what's changing around me, and where I need more self-care or support. It's incredibly supportive to see how much has changed or how much I've manifested in the six months since the new or full moon was last in the current sign. Alternatively, sometimes I discover I'm still dealing with the same issues which helps me to pivot and refocus my self-care as needed.

If you're struggling to figure out what it is that you're devoted to, ask yourself these questions and see if you can dig deep to find the answers within you:

What activities bring me the deepest sense of joy? What do I look forward to doing each day?

_____

_____

_____

During what times of the day do I feel most supported? What am I doing at those times and who am I with?

_____

_____

_____

Do I believe in any kind of a higher power? How do I express that belief?

_____

_____

_____

PUTTING IT ALL TOGETHER

Your magickal self-care practice is most likely going to consist of a combination of these internal and external forms of self-care. Achieving a natural balance of these elements will help you create a practice that deeply fulfills your own unique needs.

Taking everything you've learned in these first two chapters, do a brain dump of everything it is that you believe, all of your mental, emotional, physical, and spiritual needs as you've identified them and all the different elements of spirituality that interest you, especially in the five categories of mind, body, intuition, nature, and devotion. Check *everything* against your intuition. What resonates? What doesn't?

Although I could give you specific journal prompts here, I feel it's going to be more powerful for you to really explore this in a free-write style. Just allow yourself to be in the flow and to feel into where you have resonance in your spiritual practice. Where are the gaps? What needs are not being fulfilled right now? Ask your intuition and trust the answers you receive; no need to second-guess yourself, the answers you receive are the answers you need to hear.

In the next chapter, we're going to add one more layer to this self-care cake by taking a look at your personal astrology and learning all about how the stars can affect your needs.

Chapter 3
UNDERSTAND YOUR SELF-CARE STYLE THROUGH ASTROLOGY

Astrology is the study of the stars and how they can impact our lives and personalities. At the moment of your birth, the stars and planets were aligned in a particular pattern and this pattern can be calculated in your astrological natal chart.

When you think of astrology, you probably think of your sun sign: this is the sign that the sun was passing through at the moment you were born and the sign that you probably read your horoscope for. We can also calculate the signs of any other planet, asteroid, or celestial body, each of which is associated with a particular realm of life or aspect of your personality.

There are twelve signs in the zodiac, three signs representing each of the four elements of fire, earth, air, and water. Each planet's placement in a sign acts as a filter through which that aspect of your life appears.

When examining your self-care style and the types of self-care which will be especially nourishing for you, we are going to look at a few different celestial bodies and signs:

- Sun, because it represents your inner light and what brings you joy
- Ascendant (which denotes the eastern horizon at the moment of your birth), because it represents core aspects of your personality
- Moon, because it represents your intuitive and emotional self
- Ceres (an asteroid named for the Roman goddess of agriculture), because it represents your self-care style and the ways in which you need nourishment

We'll also be looking at the representation of the elements in your chart to see various ways which you can create balance in your life through self-care. Calculate your natal chart using an online service and then return here to read about each of your astrological placements.

To generate your astrological natal chart, you will need to know the exact date, time, and location of your birth. If you do not know the time you were born, you should disregard the ascendant sign, as you will not be able to calculate this accurately and you don't want to be looking at inaccurate information. Rather, simply calculate your chart based on an arbitrary time during the day and look at the other planets and signs suggested here.

Also, if you do not know the time you were born and the moon changed signs on your birth date, you will not be able to accurately calculate your moon sign either. In this case, your moon will be in one of two signs so feel free to read for both and follow the one that resonates with you more.

You can generate your natal chart by visiting my website www. witchoflupinehollow.com/create-your-birth-chart or your favorite online astrology site.

THE SUN AND ASCENDANT IN SELF-CARE

The sun sign represents your most intrinsic self, the part of you that shines most brightly, and the elements of life which bring you the most joy. You can think of the sun in your chart as the brightest and most buoyant of your signs. That's not to say that the sun is most important, per se. It's important to understand that your chart is most meaningful when read in a holistic way, taking into account all of your

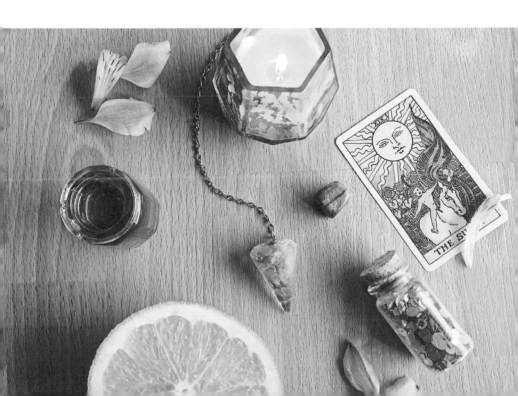

signs and the relationships between the placement of each planet. The sun has a certain brilliance about it though that draws you in.

The ascendant sign is the constellation that was rising over the eastern horizon at the moment of your birth. This sign represents the core of your personality. It's actually recommended by many astrologers to read your horoscope for your ascendant sign, not your sun sign, for greater accuracy, which goes to show you just how important this sign can be. Your ascendant is the part of you that rises up to the surface, the aspect of you that you show to the world, and that other people may be familiar with.

In terms of self-care, the sun and ascendant signs are the expressive ways you nurture yourself. Depending on your placements, this could be a creative pursuit, a type of exercise or movement, a method of communicating your needs, or an activity or interest that brings you great fulfillment and joy.

Sun or Ascendant in Aries: This placement is one of action and independence. Nurturing your inner fiery ram is about allowing yourself lots of freedom—freedom to express yourself, freedom in relationships, freedom in career, financial freedom, every kind of freedom. When Aries begins to feel trapped or held down in any way, you become irritable and aggressive. In order to nourish the fire in you, try rigorous exercise routines (essentially, sweat it out), tending to desert-loving plants like cacti, or guided meditations to clear your head, which can become full of noise.

Sun or Ascendant in Taurus: This placement is one of beauty and sensuality. Nurturing your inner earthy bull is about surrounding yourself with beauty and expressing yourself through touch. Since this is *self*-care we're talking about here, you can definitely fulfill this need by touching yourself, though exchanging platonic and romantic touch with others is also fulfilling for Taurus. When Taurus feels isolated from contact with yourself or others, you become tense and stubbornly set in your ways. In order to nourish your need for physical contact, try getting regular massages (even a chair massage at the mall will do, as will applying lotion or moisturizer with intention), walking barefoot in the grass, or wrapping yourself in a soft, cozy blanket.

Sun or Ascendant in Gemini: This placement is one of flirtatious fun. Nurturing your inner airy Gemini is about expressing yourself through words, whether written, spoken, sung, or otherwise. You love to talk (and, yes, you love a harmless flirtation), but it's rarely superficial. On the contrary, words are sacred to you and communicating your needs is a big part of self-care for you. When you feel dismissed or as though someone is not heeding your needs (and this includes a subconscious dismissal of your own needs), you become flighty and unwilling to make commitments. In order to nourish your need for open communication, try starting a regular journaling practice where you can pour out all of your thoughts onto the page without need for clarity or attend social events where you can feel free to chat and flirt as you please.

Sun or Ascendant in Cancer: This placement is one of comfort and retreat. Nurturing your inner watery crab is about allowing yourself to have the space you need. This is different than a need for freedom; rather, the needs of Cancer are around a comfortable environment and pleasant solitude. When you begin to feel over socialized or uncomfortable in a given environment, you become withdrawn and overly sensitive. In order to nourish your need for space, try setting aside a particular amount of time each day to be alone so that you can meditate, take a nap in a comfortable space you've created, or take a peaceful and restorative ritual bath. Cancer is also ruled by the moon so learning to trust your intuition is an important aspect of self-care for you.

Sun or Ascendant in Leo: This placement is one of creativity and socialization. Nurturing your inner fiery lion is about expressing yourself creatively, in whatever form that may take. Though Leos are often known as singers, actors, and public figures, this sign can also take on the form of artist, writer, comedian, or simply a natural leader of family, friends, and colleagues. When you feel stifled creatively, you become narcissistic and spend a lot of time trying to justify your worth. In order to nourish your need for creative expression, you need to determine what creative pursuits feel most fulfilling for you and then make time for them regularly. There are the traditional creative arts, of course, such as painting, acting, singing, or writing, but anything can be creative if it brings you joy. Leo is also ruled by the sun so having this placement in particular makes for a strong personality and a wise leader.

Sun or Ascendant in Virgo: This placement is one of healing and ritual. Nurturing your inner earth goddess is about owning your power. The beauty of Virgo is the complicated combination of nature-based healing practices and organization and skill-driven passions.

When you feel like you can't master something or like everything around you is in chaotic disarray, you start to try to control everyone and everything. In order to nourish your need for order, but also to honor your ability to heal yourself and others, try focusing on breathwork, an element of yourself that you have full control over if you choose to express it, tending healing herbs in an orderly garden or patio, or creating systems for your spiritual practice, such as morning and evening rituals.

Sun or Ascendant in Libra: This placement is one of balance and partnership. Nurturing your inner airy Libra is about striking balance in all areas of your life. Libra is the sign of the scales, a sign devoted to justice and fairness. When you begin to feel out of balance (such as with a poor work-life balance), or as though your values are being tested, you try to repress your own discomfort for the comfort of others, such is your ability to self-sacrifice. In order to nourish your need for balance, try creating clear boundaries around your time, especially the time you give to others.

Sun or Ascendant in Scorpio: This placement is one of magic and depth. Nurturing your inner watery scorpion is about embracing your darkness. This isn't just about your darker impulses (though Scorpio loves to explore the taboo aspects of yourself), it's also about being willing to dive deep into your dark thoughts and feelings and where they are coming from. When you feel surrounded by shallow or inauthentic people and situations, you become dismissive and cruel. In order to nourish your need for depth, try finding a divination tool that resonates with you, such as tarot cards, and using the answers you receive from your tools as a jumping-off point for deep and lengthy journal entries of self-exploration. You could also try using herbs and oils to create potions to support your needs.

Sun or Ascendant in Sagittarius: This placement is one of spirituality and adventure. Nurturing your inner fiery centaur is about getting curious. Sagittarius is obsessed with learning, educating yourself, gaining knowledge and wisdom from spiritual leaders, exploring the world, traveling to new places, and connecting with a deep source of spirit. When you feel trapped in one place or unable to have deep, meaningful conversations, you become restless and pushy. In order to nourish your need for curiosity about the world and spirituality, try spending time outside at night stargazing (as the centaur is the astrologer of the zodiac), taking regular classes on new and intriguing subjects, or practicing yoga with a focus on lingering, meditative poses.

Sun or Ascendant in Capricorn: This placement is one of stability and responsibility. Nurturing your inner earthy mountain goat is about embracing skepticism. Though you may be deeply fascinated by astrology and spirituality (as evidenced by picking up this book!), you still have some key traces of the skeptic about you. When you try to fight against your responsible, skeptical nature, you become condescending and insensitive. In order to nourish your inner skeptic, try introducing an element of critical thinking into your self-care practice: before incorporating any new concept or idea into your practice, take the time to ask yourself why it appeals to you and what aspects of it you may feel skeptical or dismissive of and why.

Sun or Ascendant in Aquarius: This placement is one of rebellion and change. Nurturing your inner airy water-bearer (an Aquarian contradiction to be sure), is about pursuing your ideals—and about being different. Sometimes Aquarius acts like it needs to be different for the sake of being different but this is more about being a leader in innovation. Whether this manifests in your life as an innovation of technology, of politics, of creative expression, or in some other way entirely, your inner Aquarius is a powerful player. When you begin to feel confined by the status quo or kept in your place by some form of authority, you become detached and unreasonable. In order to nourish your need for innovation, try using a voice recorder to record your thoughts and ideas whenever they come to you, regardless of their practical application, or join a local chapter of a political organization.

Sun or Ascendant in Pisces: This placement is one of mysticism and intuition. Nurturing your inner watery fish is about being kind to yourself. Pisces can become highly self-critical when unchecked, but you have vast potential for wisdom and intuitive insight—there's no need to be so hard on yourself! When you feel overly empathetic and zapped of energy, you become irrational and listless. In order to nourish your need for positivity, try signing up for a daily positive affirmation, listening to guided meditations for light and positivity (especially if you can do these near a body of water like the ocean, a lake, or even in the bathtub), or taking time alone to recharge your batteries and reset your empathic abilities.

THE MOON IN SELF-CARE

The moon represents your intuitive and emotional self. These are two distinct aspects so let's take them each in turn. Your intuitive moon sign shows you what kinds of tools are going to be supportive for you in nurturing your intuition, as well as the ways in which you receive intuitive downloads and your natural ability to trust your intuition. Because intuition is such a nebulous thing, each of us receives, processes, and trusts it in a different way, and your moon sign can provide insight into your unique intuitive perspective.

Your emotional moon is all about the ways in which you feel, what makes you get emotional, how you express your emotions, and how you perceive the emotions of others. Intuition and emotions are inextricably linked, as allowing yourself to "feel the feels" is one of the key elements of really tapping into your intuition. Allowing

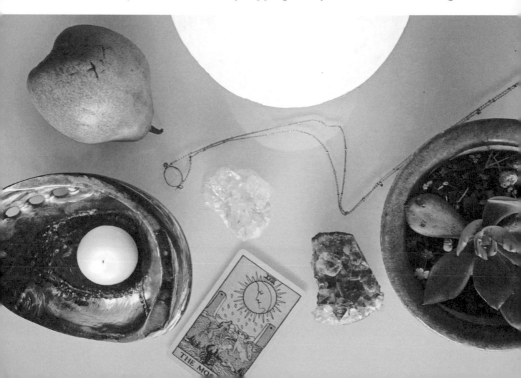

yourself to get raw and emotional will guide you in deepening and strengthening your trust in your intuition and make you more open to receiving those intuitive hits.

In terms of self-care, your moon sign provides a window into what your soul needs. Where the sun and ascendant are more external and active pursuits, the moon is about your internal landscape. This is where you can dive deep into the forms of self-care that go beyond the bubble bath: we're talking about emotional, mental, and spiritual nourishment.

Moon in Aries: This placement is one of distraction and aggression. Intuitively, Aries can feel at odds with the watery and flowing energy of the moon. Aries wants to rush forward, headlong, but intuition requires taking the time to stop and listen to yourself—and a certain willingness to follow the guidance of your intuition instead of your head or ego. Aries is often dismissive of your own emotions and those of others, but can become bent out of shape when your emotions are dismissed by others. In order to trust your intuition, make meditation a regular part of your routine so that you begin spending time listening to yourself—listening to your breath, your heartbeat, and your intuition. To nourish your emotional needs, you need to really allow yourself to let those aggressive emotions out. When you're angry, sad, or frustrated, tell someone or write it down. Better yet, as Aries is more of a doer than a talker, find a place you can be alone and scream it out!

Moon in Taurus: This placement is one of grounded energy. Intuitively, Taurus is very connected to the body. You receive your intuitive hits in the physical realm. You might be susceptible to illness, especially when you are feeling anxious or unaligned with something. You can feel it in your bones when something is or is not right for you. Emotionally, you also process internal information in the physical—you might become ill or injured when you are trying to hold in your emotions. To nourish your emotional needs, find the places on your body where you really hold onto things. This might be your shoulders or shoulder blades, hips, feet, etc.—likely the place where you most often feel tense or tight. Practice breathing into this space and releasing tension, especially just prior to or after a deep journaling or meditation session.

Moon in Gemini: This placement is one of mental acuity and communication. You process intuitive downloads and emotions through words, either writing or speaking. This may depend on the phase your moon sign is in: waxing signs are more likely to be speakers and more outgoing, while waning signs are more likely to be writers and more introverted. Intuitively, you may find that practices such as automatic writing are well-suited to you, where you simply pour your thoughts out onto the page for a given amount of time. When you read back over them, you may be surprised to discover how much wisdom you already had. To nourish your emotional needs, you always need to talk it out, whether with a friend or loved one or even a therapist or life coach. Even talking to the mirror can help you process sometimes!

Moon in Cancer: This placement is one of deep emotional waters. The moon is at home in Cancer, so this combination makes for a strong sense of intuition and emotional expression. All forms of divination and intuitive techniques are likely to work for you, but you will probably find as you explore the different options that there are one or two in particular that really give you the most accurate results. You may be accused of being overly sensitive and emotional at times, but this sensitivity is actually one of your greatest strengths. You are highly attuned to the emotional needs of others, making you very caring and perhaps even empathic. To nourish your own emotional needs though, as it's very important in such a sensitive person to not favor the needs of others over your own, you may very well need to retreat regularly so that you can rest and reset as needed.

Moon in Leo: This placement is one of wisdom and sovereignty. The aspect of Leo that gets all the attention is that of the bold, brash, and flamboyant performer. It's often noted that many actors and singers are Leo suns. But Leo is also the wise Lion, sovereign of the jungle. Intuitively, this may come through in the form of innate knowing, also called claircognizance, a clear sense of simply knowing the answer. You may experience dramatic displays of emotion or you may really bottle up your emotions and only show your hand when you so choose; this may depend on your moon phase with the waxing Leo moon displaying emotions and the waning Leo moon hiding them. To nourish your emotional needs, take the opportunity whenever you can to really shine the light of the sun on them and try to look at your emotional self objectively. Leo is ruled by the sun and this placement can really help you balance out the watery energy of the moon and fiery energy of the sun.

Moon in Virgo: This placement is one of organized thought and self-healing. Virgo loves to organize and although this need for a neat and orderly life can be at odds with the messiness of trusting your intuition and expressing your emotions, you can absolutely embrace this placement's differences. Tarot journaling or another form of documenting your intuitive experiments will serve you well, giving you an opportunity to get in touch with your intuition in a tangible way. Emotionally, Virgo needs to feel the satisfaction of self-healing. As a powerful healer, Virgo is wonderful at healing others through grounding and connecting to the earth's energy, but in order to nourish your emotional needs, be sure to turn those talents on yourself on a regular basis as well.

Moon in Libra: This placement is one of mediation and discussion. Because Libra is all about balance, you dislike expressing messy emotions, but you are excellent at helping others work through their own. You often feel as though expressing your emotions will damage your relationships, as you never like to upset the people you care about (or even strangers). This diplomacy can keep you in a gridlock if you let it overtake you, but it can also serve you well in that you are able to look objectively at your own feelings and at those of others and begin to see where your thinking may be flawed. Being able to see flaws in this manner is a form of intuition in and of itself, as not everyone is gifted with this talent of objectivity.

Moon in Scorpio: This placement is one of deep psychic ability and torrential emotions. Scorpio feels everything very deeply, so your emotions may sometimes threaten to control you. That very feeling of overwhelm can make you feel even more emotional (in whatever manner you are currently expressing, such as sadness or anger), as Scorpio hates to feel out of control or at the mercy of someone or something. This is one of your greatest strengths though, not a weakness at all. The depth of your emotions is powerful, if you allow yourself to feel it, and to embrace even the emotions you have been taught to see as "dark." It's okay to be sad, it's okay to be angry, as long as you have a self-awareness around those emotions and do the inner work to process through them. As for intuition, Scorpio has the ability to tap into the collective in spades. Scorpio is one of the witchiest signs and is heavily associated with the occult, so divination tools such as tarot and runes will serve you well.

Moon in Sagittarius: This placement is one of spiritual enlightenment and wanderlust. Sagittarius has a very difficult time sitting still, so sitting with your emotions and being present with yourself can be a challenge, as you always want to be on the move—even on the move from your own feelings. Try taking the time to be really still and quiet on a regular basis and allow yourself to listen to your own needs and express the feelings you may be holding in subconsciously. You feel most tuned in to your intuition when you are traveling—being surrounded by the hustle and bustle of the city (likely a waxing moon trait), or vast, expansive wilderness (a waning moon trait), makes you feel connected and alert.

Moon in Capricorn: This placement can be a tense one, as Capricorn is the opposite sign of Cancer, the home sign of the moon. That doesn't have to be a negative or a weakness though—in fact, this combination represents the divine masculine and divine feminine at balance. Though listening to and trusting your intuition may not come very naturally to you, if you devote yourself to this process and allow your skepticism to guide you, you will become highly attuned to what truly resonates. That innate skepticism will keep you solidly planted on the right path for you, as long as you don't allow it to control your choices either. Expressing emotions can be a tense experience for Capricorn as well. Though Capricorn is a feminine earth sign, it's also ruled by the authoritative, father-figure energy of Saturn. Embrace this study in opposites to create a deeply supportive (divine feminine) and sustainable (divine masculine) self-care practice.

Moon in Aquarius: This placement is one of reason and logic. Aquarius truly values debate and finding solutions, so overt emotion can feel like a waste of time, which is why Aquarians are often accused of being too detached. But "logicking" your way through emotions can be a positive experience when done with intention and awareness. Take the opportunity to look at your own feelings from a higher perspective: why are you feeling what you're feeling, and what solutions can you find for yourself? When handling the emotions of other people though, do try not to be too much of a "fixer." Sometimes our loved ones just want an ear, not a problem-solver. Intuitively, Aquarius just knows what is *right*. Having a profound sense of right and wrong, you have no difficulty following the right path for you and encouraging others to join you.

Moon in Pisces: This placement is one of empathy and wisdom. You feel emotions on a soul level and can empathically pick up on the feelings of others. In some cases, this can lead to depression, obsessiveness, and addictions, as Pisces tries desperately to hide from the onslaught of emotion. Being an empathetic person is a wondrous gift, though, if you set healthy boundaries around the way others share their feelings with you (since you are a magnet for this), and around the way you allow the energy of others to merge with your own. Pisces is considered the "eldest" sign in the zodiac, the sign which has progressed through all of its karmic cycles and learned all of its lessons, so there is deep wisdom here. Your intuition is all-encompassing and information comes to you in a variety of ways. This can be overwhelming at times but taking quiet moments to allow your intuitive downloads to come through can be very powerful.

CERES: THE ASTEROID OF SELF-CARE

While the sun and moon and the other planets in our solar system represent aspects of who you are, there are literally tens of thousands of other celestial bodies which we can also plot on our natal chart. Many of these are somewhat inconsequential, given the vast number of stars, asteroids, and other bodies in our galaxy. However, some asteroids have been found to have a deeply nuanced impact on the natal chart and can be well-worth charting. The asteroid Ceres was discovered in 1801 in the asteroid belt between Mars and Jupiter. It is so large that in 2006, scientists actually reclassified it as a dwarf planet, although astrologers typically consider this celestial body one of the "goddess asteroids" which gives us a unique perspective on specific areas of life.

Ceres is named for the Greek goddess of fertility and agriculture. In

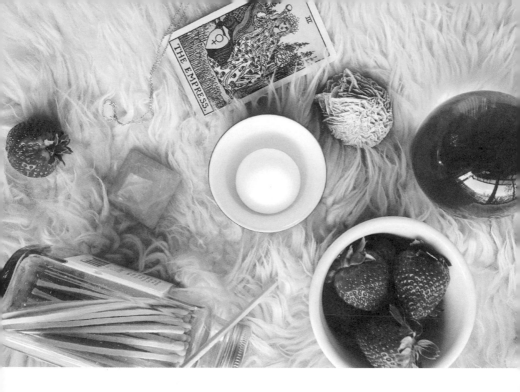

Rome, she was known as Demeter, and is the mother of Persephone, the goddess of spring who became Queen of the Underworld and wife of the god, Hades. It is said that Persephone descends into the Underworld to be with her husband each year for six months, during which time her mother grieves and all crops wither and die. Come spring, Persephone returns to her mother and the fields become fertile once more as Ceres/Demeter rejoices in her resurrection. For this reason, Ceres represents abundance, fertility, and growth but also motherhood, grief, and nurturance.

One of the reasons that Ceres and the other goddess asteroids (Pallas, Juno, and Vesta) are such powerful, if somewhat obscure, signs to look at in your astrological natal chart is because of the general lack of "feminine" planets. All of the planets in our solar system except Venus are named for male gods. Though half of the zodiac signs are considered "feminine" (those ruled by the earth and water elements), the planets do not have the same equality, so the goddess asteroids balance out that mythological oversight. In astrology, the concepts of masculine and feminine do not indicate male or female, but rather archetypal experiences that we all have, regardless of gender.

In modern-day astrology, the dwarf planet, Ceres, is considered the asteroid of self-care. At its root, the concept of self-care is an archetypally feminine one—the practice of nurturing ourselves, caring for our needs, allowing ourselves to be emotional, sensitive beings with very human wounds and shadows. (Although in later chapters, we'll be exploring the need for divine masculine archetypes in your self-care practice as well!)

Your Ceres sign represents the root of your need for self-care. This is the area of your life in which you need the most support, nourishment, and grounding energy. Most importantly, this is where you must learn to care for *yourself*. Support from others in this area of your life may feel extra nourishing, but only if you have already learned to nourish yourself in that way first. That's the thing about self-care: it can come from many sources but external self-care is only effective when we understand why we need it. Ceres is also about doing the shadow work and processing your traumas. As Ceres/Demeter grieved the loss of her daughter each year, so do we all experience some kind of grief. Self-care is not just about bubble baths and pampering yourself; it's also about meeting your shadows and learning to live together, as Ceres and Hades learned to share the love of Persephone.

Ceres in Aries: This placement is one of active self-care. You need to really step up for yourself and make it happen—otherwise, your needs may fall through the cracks and go untended until it is no longer sustainable. It is all too easy for Aries not to worry about taking care of the inner work: Aries wants to spend all the time in your head or out doing all of the things, but you often forget or even willfully ignore your internal needs. If confronting your shadows makes you want to run into the brightest, sunniest room you can find and hide from that internal darkness . . . well, you might be an Aries. To truly fulfill your self-care needs, you need to take an active role in confronting those shadows and in scheduling time to express and care for your emotional needs. These emotional needs are not a weakness, but rather an opportunity to stoke your inner fire.

Ceres in Taurus: This placement is one of sensual self-care. As the goddess of agriculture and fertility, Ceres has a naturally earthy quality and Taurus is the fixed earth sign of the zodiac so these two together make for a profoundly grounded experience. You definitely require physical self-care, including massage and comfortable surroundings and spending time in nature, but your Ceres placement also suggests that you really need to express your sensuality. You may well have some shadows around allowing yourself to be sensual, whether alone, with a partner, or even in public. You need to nourish this side of yourself and embrace your sensual nature.

Ceres in Gemini: This placement is one of expressive self-care. One of the tenets of your self-care practice is the need to express your needs! You must nourish your voice, as Gemini is the communicator of the zodiac. Speaking up for yourself, communicating your needs to those around you, and expressing your needs within your own self-care practice are vital to your overall well-being. This certainly includes communicating with yourself, taking the time to stop and listen to what your mind, body, and heart have to say.

Ceres in Cancer: This placement is one of intuitive self-care. Cancer is the sign of the moon and is deeply connected to your intuition. You need to nourish your connection to your inner knowing and wisdom and pay close attention to the cycles of your body and emotions. You may find that you are affected more than others by the phases of the moon and that your needs wax and wane with the phases as well. Tracking your energy levels and what kinds of self-care you feel drawn to may prove very insightful for you. For example, you may feel more active and want to exercise or be social during the waxing phase of the moon while the waning phase may bring a more introverted need for self-reflection and alone time. Be sure to check in with yourself on a regular basis and ask your intuition what your needs are and how you can meet them.

Ceres in Leo: This placement is one of creative self-care. Leo needs play in your life, a sense of creative fun and letting loose. You need to nourish your creativity and the activities that get you in touch with your inner child. This can express itself in any number of ways, whether it be writing, painting, drawing, singing, acting, or anything else that makes you feel like a kid again and allows you to really express your creative spark. Being around children may also activate this part of yourself, so playing with your own kids or making time to teach or volunteer at a school or day care could be a really nourishing experience for you.

Ceres in Virgo: This placement is one of sacred self-care. Virgo is represented by the Virgin, a symbol and archetype often associated with ancient priestesses, such as the Vestal Virgins of Rome. You need to embrace and nurture the sacred priestess within you. Creating sacred spaces is going to be deeply nourishing for you. That could look like anything from decorating your bedroom and private spaces with care to setting up altars to your self-care practice or to a deity or something else that is sacred to you. You define what sacredness means to you.

Ceres in Libra: This placement indicates the need to be selfish sometimes. Libra can be a truly selfless and self-sacrificing sign, always trying to be as diplomatic and balanced as possible, keeping the peace between loved ones, coworkers, and friends. That responsibility which you have placed on yourself can become a burden if you do not sometimes remove the mantle and allow yourself to be selfish. First, though, you probably need to do some shadow work around what exactly the words selfless and selfish mean to you! Do some journaling or meditating around these words and how they appear in your life. What does it mean to be selfish and how can you give that word a positive connotation? When does being selfless have a negative connotation?

Ceres in Scorpio: This placement is one of shadow work. Of all the signs, Scorpio is the most dedicated to doing shadow work and getting deep with yourself. Depth, authenticity, and having the tough conversations, even internally, are all part of Scorpio's wheelhouse. You need to get comfortable with being uncomfortable and find the shadow aspects of yourself that need to be addressed. This is an ongoing process, not a one-and-done experience, so expect to find new shadows just as soon as you feel the last have been processed.

Ceres in Sagittarius: This placement is one of spiritual self-care. Sagittarius craves spiritual connection and enlightenment. You need to nourish your need for wisdom and education, for exploration of parts unknown, including the unknown aspects of yourself. Take time for self-reflection and to educate yourself about anything and everything that interests you, especially of a spiritual nature. You need depth of understanding of the topics that appeal to you; make sure you hold yourself accountable for follow-through and for getting deep with yourself.

Ceres in Capricorn: This placement is one of grounded self-care. Capricorn needs stability and to feel as though you are capable of standing on your own two feet. You value self-sufficiency and responsibility and that carries over into your self-care practice. Though Capricorn can be a skeptical and stoic sign, the ability to support and nourish yourself comes quite naturally, flowing from the divine masculine. Grounding activities such as grounding meditations, earthing (the act of walking barefoot on soil or grass), and simply feeling into and becoming aware of your physical body will be very nourishing for you, as will any activities that allow you to express your responsibility for your own well-being.

Ceres in Aquarius: This placement indicates the need for self-care so that you can accomplish great things. As the humanitarian of the zodiac, Aquarius is often associated with political and human rights activism, or other forms of giving back to the community and the collective. With Ceres in Aquarius, you need to make time for yourself so that you can affect the great changes you see must be made around you. As they say, you can't pour from an empty cup, and taking the time to fill your own cup through acts of self-care will open you up to the many possibilities of the Age of Aquarius.

Ceres in Pisces: This placement is one of learning to trust. As the last sign in the zodiac, Pisces is flowing with the wisdom of the ancestors and all the signs before it. Deeply connected to your intuition, you must learn to trust your inner voice for it contains all the wisdom of the universe. Pisces self-care is about learning to trust yourself but also learning to trust the infinite unknown. Divination tools will serve you well, but I also recommend time for quiet self-reflection, just listening to your inner voice and allowing it to speak through you with love.

CREATING BALANCE WITH THE ELEMENTS

Each sign is associated with one of the four elements: fire, earth, air, and water. Fire and air are considered active, "masculine" energies, while earth and water are considered intuitive, "feminine" energies, each with their own expression of that:

- **Fire (Aries, Leo, Sagittarius):** The most active element, representing action, creativity, and movement

- **Earth (Taurus, Virgo, Capricorn):** The most grounded element, representing comfort, stability, and abundance
- **Air (Gemini, Libra, Aquarius):** The most intellectual element, representing thought, ideas, and abstractions
- **Water (Cancer, Scorpio, Pisces):** The most intuitive element, representing emotions, depth, and wisdom

For even greater nuance, each sign within an element represents a unique expression of those energies. For example, Taurus, Virgo, and Capricorn are all earth signs. Earth signs all have a certain grounded physicality and affinity for nature, but each sign expresses this a bit differently. Taurus is very connected to the sensual body and comforts, Virgo is connected to healing talents and plants, and Capricorn has an affinity for the successes and goals of the material world.

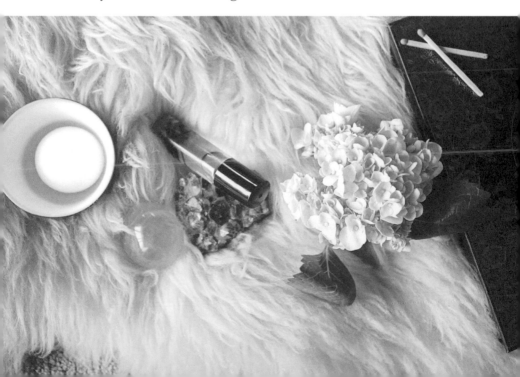

As you look through your chart and your unique placements of the planets in signs, you will likely notice that some signs have several planets in them and others may be completely empty of planets. Those signs that hold multiple planets in your chart are called a stellium, a cluster of planets in a single sign. This creates a strong energetic signature of that sign's expression within you. The same goes for the elements. When you have a cluster of planets in any one element, you express the energies of that element more strongly than the others. When you have no or very few planets in any one element, you express those energies very little in your life and may have a difficult time relating to those energies in others.

Though some people have a fairly even distribution of planets across the elements, it's common to have an elemental imbalance in your chart. Addressing that imbalance isn't about "fixing" yourself, as there are really no bad astrological placements. You may hear scary things about retrograde planets, solar and lunar eclipses, "bad" signs, or challenging aspects, but all of these concepts within astrology are there to teach you more about yourself, so that you can learn and grow. Even the greatest challenges you might find in your chart are there for your benefit, a lesson written in the stars for you to learn over the course of a lifetime.

When you do have an elemental imbalance, though, it can create an imbalance in your self-care practice as well. Incorporating aspects of the elements which you have very little of in your chart, as well as honoring the elements you have strong placements in, will strengthen your self-care practice and make it even more supportive of your actual needs.

Look at your entire natal chart and make note of how many planets (including ascendant and asteroids), you have positioned in each of the elements.

- # of Planets in Fire Signs: _____
- # of Planets in Earth Signs: _____
- # of Planets in Air Signs: _____
- # of Planets in Water Signs: _____

Any element which you have four or more planets placed in is a strong placement. Any element which you have two or fewer planets placed in is a minor placement, where you are expressing those elements very little.

Strong Placement in Fire: If you have a strong fire placement, you likely feel very driven. You have a deep need for action and movement in your life and have a clear vision of what you desire. You may be prone to emotional outbursts of temper or arrogance. In your self-care practice, consider incorporating more watery elements to balance out this strong fire energy. Take cooling baths, drink iced teas (especially with cooling herbs like mint), and spend time in quiet, peaceful spaces. This isn't about calming or taming your inner fire, but rather about directing your focus and giving yourself the space to be emotional when need be. When out of balance, fire has a tendency to burn hot and wild—and to burn out quickly. Embracing the opposite element of water will help to balance this internal wildfire.

Minor Placement in Fire: If you have a minor fire placement, with two or fewer planets or asteroids in fire signs, you may feel very emotional, steadfast, or head-in-the-clouds, depending on which elements you have the most of in your chart. Regardless of your other planetary placements, try incorporating fiery self-care practices into your life to activate this part of yourself. Though your action-oriented, inner warrior may be lying dormant, that doesn't mean you can't rouse them when needed. Find ways to fire yourself up, whether it be through strenuous exercise, vigorous debate, or even literally spending time in warm places.

Strong Placement in Earth: If you have a strong earth placement, you likely feel very grounded. You have a strong desire for stability, efficiency, and pleasure in your life. You may have a tendency to become stuck in a rut or stick stubbornly with a decision, long after it's been proven to be the wrong choice. In your self-care practice, consider incorporating more airy elements to balance out this strong earth energy. Air is all about the vast, open expanse of the mind. Spend time in intellectual pursuits, especially studying abstract concepts (like astrology!), and get comfortable being in your head. You spend a lot of your life feeling everything in your physical body; release your grip a bit and allow yourself to dream and imagine.

Minor Placement in Earth: If you have a minor earth placement, with two or fewer planets or asteroids in earth signs, you may feel very adrift and ungrounded, untethered to the earth, and disconnected from your body, depending on which elements you have the most of in your chart. Regardless of your other planetary placements, try incorporating earthy self-care practices into your life to activate this part of yourself. Touch is the most important sense for the earth element, so try getting massages or just touching yourself with intention, paying attention to the physical sensations of being a human having an earthly experience. Spend time in nature, as well, connecting with the literal earth and feeling the grass or dirt beneath your feet.

Strong Placement in Air: If you have a strong air placement, you likely feel very, well, up in the air. You have many diverse interests and are often pursuing multiple ideas at once. You may struggle with follow-through as you're easily distracted. In your self-care practice, consider incorporating more earthy elements to balance out this strong air energy. Earth is the most grounded of the signs and will help bring you back down to reality when you've drifted away. This isn't about tethering you or keeping you from exploring, but rather about giving you a place to land when you need to. Even the most adventuresome need a place to call home. Create some sacred spaces where you can rest and get out of your head when you feel the need.

Minor Placement in Air: If you have a minor air placement, with two or fewer planets or asteroids in air signs, you may struggle to find the inspiration you need in order to best express your other elements. Regardless of your other planetary placements, try incorporating airy self-care practices into your life to activate this part of yourself. Create art or beauty in whatever way feels good to you and spend time in intellectual study on any topic that you find interesting. Allow yourself to meditate, journal, and connect with your higher self to find your sources of inspiration.

Strong Placement in Water: If you have a strong water placement, you likely feel very connected to your emotions and intuition. You feel things more deeply than other people and you express your emotions more readily. You may be prone to bouts of depression or sadness, though you are also capable of feeling effusive joy. In your self-care practice, consider incorporating more fiery elements to balance out this strong water energy. Allow yourself to get mad and to express that. Find the things in life that make your heart beat faster or that scare you just a little and jump into them, feet first. This isn't about ignoring your intuition or tamping down your emotional expression, as those abilities are both incredible gifts. Incorporating fire into your life is about keeping you from getting waterlogged and bogged down by the depth of feeling that you experience.

Minor Placement in Water: If you have a minor water placement, with two or fewer planets or asteroids in water signs, you may struggle to express your emotions or to get in touch with and trust your intuition. Regardless of your other planetary placements, try incorporating watery self-care practices into your life to activate this part of yourself. Divination tools and dream journaling will help you get in touch with your intuitive side, while ritual bathing and visiting the ocean will connect you with the relaxing sound and sensation of water itself. Also allow yourself to get emotional and to really feel your emotions. Tap in and let yourself cry when you need to.

Astrology is an incredibly powerful tool for learning to understand yourself better. This is where your self-care practice truly begins, with understanding who you truly are. Often, we think we know who we are and what we need, but we're actually acting out a script that's been written for us by our ancestors, parents, friends, teachers, bosses, and coworkers and the expectations each of them has put on us (whether intentionally or not).

Astrology does not tell you your fate or destiny, nor does it predict when you're going to get married or promoted. Astrology is a language of energy that gives you a road map of who you *could* be, of the person you could *choose* to express, and of your natural tendencies for certain behaviors, desires, and modes of expression. When you begin to learn to speak this language and interpret it in your own life, you discover the scripts you've been following that don't actually resonate with you on a soul level. Maybe you've been following the responsible, expected path in your career (a strong expression of the earth element), but secretly, have always wanted to quit your job and make a living bungee jumping (definitely a fire element desire!). Come to find out you have an abundance of fire in your chart and a Sagittarius sun . . . time to embrace who you really are and step out of the script that's been handed to you!

That's an extreme example, of course, but many of us are acting out of the desire to fulfill our obligations and to meet the expectations of those we care about. Those are noble goals and you don't have to ditch your duty in order to start practicing magickal, transformative self-care, but no one ever experienced soulful transformation by sticking with the status quo.

Look at your chart for inspiration in crafting your self-care practice and then ask yourself: What actually resonates with me? What makes me feel nourished, cared for, alive, and free?

Chapter 4
CRAFT YOUR OWN
SELF-CARE RITUALS

We've spent the first section of this book learning to understand your unique self-care style. As you've learned, your personal astrology is a big factor as well as your lifestyle, mental and physical health, and your own spiritual and recreational interests. In the next few chapters, we're going to learn how to implement that style in your life by crafting meaningful self-care rituals, which are many and varied. There are as many forms of witchy self-care rituals as there are, well, witches! That's why it's so important to create your own instead of just copying those you see in books and on blogs.

The last section of this book, starting with Chapter 7 on page 144, includes rituals to inspire you but, here's the thing, inspiration is just one-third of invention, as they say. If you find a ritual written down somewhere that really resonates with you, really checks off all your boxes and that feels nourishing and fulfilling of your own unique needs . . . then by all means, do it! And if you find a ritual that doesn't quite check off all the boxes but parts of it feel right . . . then take the parts that work and leave those that don't. Most importantly, if you come across a ritual in this book or in any other that doesn't feel right *at all* or makes your intuition flare up with an instant "no," then *don't do that ritual.* This goes for every kind of ritual, spell, and magickal working. Asking your intuition what's right for you and trusting the answers you receive is absolutely paramount in witchcraft and even more so when it comes to self-care, as this is a path that is literally about your*self*. Remember that no one else's ritual is designed to fulfill your needs specifically.

In particular, I want to be sure that you protect yourself from falling into the rut of thinking that you need to do someone else's ritual because of any of the following reasons:

- You don't think you know enough to be able to create your own rituals.
- You don't think you have been studying or practicing long enough to be able to create your own rituals.
- You don't think you're a good enough or experienced enough witch to be able to create your own rituals.

All of those "reasons" are just doubt, fear, and negative self-talk trying to sway you from the path of your highest potential. Because when you're living in alignment with your intuition and taking the time for meaningful self-care, you don't need to know anything from any book, this one included. The only thing you need to "know" to be able to create your own rituals is that you know yourself and you know how to listen to your own needs!

Now that we have that cleared up, let's dive right in and talk about the anatomy of a self-care ritual.

ANATOMY OF A SELF-CARE RITUAL: PURPOSE

First of all, what is the purpose of your self-care practice? Obviously, it is to care for yourself, but what is the deeper purpose?

I think the purpose of my own self-care practice, and perhaps of the collective pursuit of self-care as well, is to find balance. Balance of the elements and balance of the divine masculine and divine feminine. These concepts of divinity are not really specific to gender, but are rather archetypes that helps us to understand the energy of everything around us. Most of us are "too in our divine masculine" or "too in our divine feminine," meaning we are embracing an imbalance of energies within ourselves. The divine masculine is all things structured, foundational, and firm. The divine feminine is all things intuitive, flowing, and changeable.

A truly balanced self-care practice incorporates both energies. You might think that self-care is inherently feminine, but a practice that only relies on the divine feminine and flowing with your intuition may be difficult to stick to, with no roots to keep you grounded. I often hear from my clients that they are resistant to creating specific self-care rituals because they don't want to be hemmed in; they want to be able to flow with their intuition. The answer to this puzzle is to balance the energies of the divine masculine and divine feminine. Self-care *is* inherently an expression of the divine feminine, of trusting your intuition and nurturing yourself. However, without a foundation of logic and structure, your practice will be ultimately unsustainable. Your intuitive, feminine self-care practice also needs an equal and opposite expression of the divine masculine to root it in reality. Striking that balance is the key to supportive *and* sustainable spiritual self-care. In this chapter, we'll be applying the need for structure to all of the intuitive information you've gathered about yourself throughout this book so far, to create self-care rituals that are supportive and sustainable for you.

Okay, then, so what is the purpose of an individual self-care ritual within your practice?

The definition of a ritual is a series of acts, especially with religious or spiritual significance, that are performed according to a prescribed order. That's not really *our* definition of a ritual for the purposes of this book, but it is good to keep in mind that rituals are a series of acts that you get to prescribe the meaning and order of. Consistency and repetition are hallmarks of traditional rituals, which you can ascribe to, or not. It's entirely up to you. Asking yourself why you're doing something or why you want something can be so powerful. Often, we move through life, making decisions and acting on certain desires, without ever really questioning *why*. But, just as every three-year-old knows, "why" is the most important and valuable question we can ask. As we grow older, we stop asking the incessant "why" questions of our toddler years, which is really a shame, because it's an absolutely vital part of developing a fulfilling self-care practice as an adult. As you do this internal work of learning how to nurture yourself, you will be so guided and supported by reclaiming your inner child and getting truly curious about your own motivations, desires, and shadows.

So, let me ask the question in a slightly different way: What is the purpose of a self-care ritual, for *you*?

Determining focus and purpose in your spiritual practice in general will give you so much more fulfillment in the long run. Tapping into your personal astrology and finding what resonates with you is the first step in creating a practice that feels exciting and nourishing but it's a continual process. This isn't something you can expect to do just once and instantly have a practice that will be fulfilling for you throughout your life; expect your needs and desires to shift with time. So, as you create your morning and evening rituals and experiment with the other rituals in this book, be sure you are continually asking yourself what it is you are drawn to and, always, *why*. On the other hand, also be sure you are remaining open-minded, now and always. Often, a practice that wasn't right for you in the past, reappears in a new way and is suddenly the doorway to a whole new perspective. Being closed off to that practice because it wasn't right in the past could keep you closed off to new perspectives and opportunities.

As you determine the purpose of your self-care practice, you'll discover specific needs that arise, which can often be fulfilled by particular rituals. A few examples of the purpose of your self-care practice could include:

- A need to step away from your busy life to avoid burnout and relieve stress
- A desire to feel spiritually connected to something larger than yourself
- A calling to connect with your intuition so that it can support you in all areas of life

By creating rituals designed to fulfill specific needs that are unique to you, you're going to be creating a spiritual and self-care practice that is not only sustainable but a vital part of your well-being. And, remember that those needs will change over time so this is not a one-and-done process!

The first piece of the anatomy of a self-care ritual is the foundation. What are the specific needs that this ritual is meant to fulfill? Depending on the purpose of your practice, you will have certain specific needs that you need to create rituals to fulfill. Addressing the first example above, a self-care practice serving a need to step away from your busy life to avoid burnout and relieve stress, here are a few potential and very specific needs that could be fulfilled by ritual:

- A need to stop yourself from diving straight into work as soon as you get up in the morning could be fulfilled by creating a morning ritual that involves no technology and no checking work emails before a certain time
- A need to take time and space in solitude, even away from your family, for at least a few minutes every day could be fulfilled by creating an evening ritual in which you disconnect and go to bed ten minutes before your partner so you can have time for meditation and reading

Notice how we're not trying to create a single ritual that serves the rather broad purpose of avoiding burnout and relieving stress. Self-care is not something you can assign ten minutes of your day to and then forget about. (It's also not something you have to devote unreasonable and unsustainable amounts of time to either . . . see Chapter 6 on page 123 for more on this.)

By choosing clear and specific changes you want to create in your life, you can direct the energy of the ritual intentionally. Ask yourself what you want to get out of this ritual as you're creating it. Does that sound selfish or crass to you? If so, I would invite you to then ask yourself why you have that reaction. Self-care is not selfish and it's not selfish to want to know what you get out of your own self-care either. It's easy to pursue a spiritual path without a clear intention because you think you're just supposed to want a vague sense of fulfillment or an undefined idea of enlightenment. The reality is that you engage with your spirituality because you want something: you want to create a better, more comfortable life or you want to experience support from within and without or you want to get to know yourself or the divine more deeply.

The burnout- and stress-focused ritual examples I've given above showcase the importance of creating rituals that serve a particular function. Identifying the purpose of your individual rituals is so important to creating them in a way that is sustainable and nourishing; just imagine what defining the purpose of your self-care practice as a whole or even your entire spiritual path could do for you.

ANATOMY OF A SELF-CARE RITUAL: FIVE PILLARS OF DIVINITY

The second aspect of the anatomy of a self-care ritual is structure. What are the actual components that make up your ritual? In the system I've created, which we touched on in Chapter 2 on page 46, there are five basic pillars of all rituals, what I like to call the Pillars of Divinity: mind, body, nature, divination/intuition, and devotion. Some, but not all, rituals include all five components, but you really only need one for any activity to become a ritual. Pretty much any activity you could incorporate into a ritual falls into one or more of these five categories.

Mind rituals encompass anything that takes place primarily in your psyche, such as the less physical senses of sight, smell, and sound. Anything that engages your mental faculties such as meditation or journaling. Even breathwork can be a form of mind ritual.

Body rituals are all about your physical experience. The physical senses of taste and touch come into play here, so any ritual that involves consuming food or drink would be appropriate, as would engaging the sense of touch through bathing, soft fabrics, sensual clothing, and massage. Movement is also a form of body ritual so anything that asks you to move your body is perfect, from yoga to dance to having sex.

Nature rituals involve anything that gives us access to the power of Mother Nature. This is perhaps the broadest category, because any activity that helps you to engage with the natural world can fall here. Gardening and hiking are obvious options, but herbalism, stargazing, and earthing (walking barefoot on the earth) are also great examples.

Divination rituals are those most mystical activities that honor and nourish our intuition. Whether you are literally trying to divine the future or just learning to trust your intuition, divination tools range from tarot and oracle cards to tea leaves to runes to pendulums and more. Perhaps the deepest and most powerful form of divination is simply sitting in quiet meditation and asking yourself: what do I need to know?

Finally, devotional rituals are perhaps the most difficult of these categories to pin down but have the greatest potential for depth of personal growth. Devotionals are any activity which expresses your devotion to something you deeply believe in. It is common to express devotion to a deity through offerings or prayer but most of

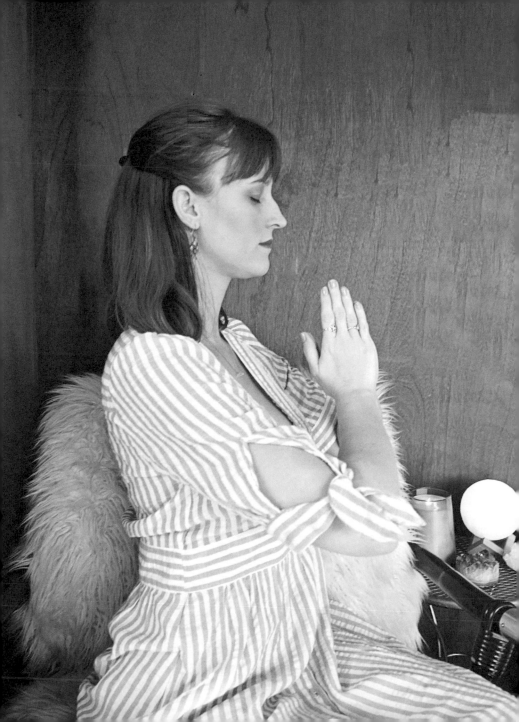

us are devoted at least as much to our families or beliefs as we are to a god, if not more. Your spiritual practice should not be a separate entity from the rest of your life, and expressing devotion to the ideas that are most important to you is a powerful way to tie your "magickal" and "mundane" lives together. Examples include creating art, cooking food for your loved ones, or political activism.

The beauty of these categories is in the ways they overlap and fit together as many activities fall into more than one category. For example, tea rituals could represent the mind, for the meditative experience of brewing and sipping tea. They could represent the body, for the physical consumption of tea, potentially made from healing plants and herbs. They could represent nature, for the plants used to brew the tea itself. They could represent divination, if you incorporate the art of tasseography, reading the tea leaves. Or they could even represent devotion, if you are giving the tea as an offering to your deity or even to your loved ones.

Depending on your purpose and focus, these five Pillars of Divinity can become stretched and expanded in any way you need them to be. Here are some examples of each. Note the overlaps!

Mind:
- Journaling, including nature, tarot, and dream journaling
- Meditation
- Aromatherapy
- Coloring books
- Listening to and making music

Body:

- Yoga and stretching
- Cardio exercise
- Sexuality and sex magick
- Working with the menstrual cycle
- Bathing
- Massage and spa services
- Skin care and makeup
- Meditating with crystals (in the hands or on the body)
- Cooking, eating, and drinking

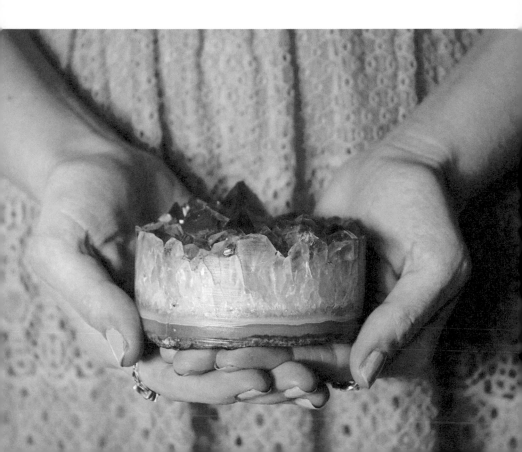

Nature:

- Spending time outside
- Gardening
- Nature journaling
- Working with herbs for healing or cooking
- Working with crystals for healing or inspiration
- Working with the seasons
- Stargazing and working with astrology

Divination/Intuition:

- Tarot and oracle cards
- Runes
- Pendulums
- Scrying
- Tasseography
- Palmistry
- Dream and tarot journaling

Devotional:

- Working with deities, spirits, or other entities
- Reading and notating in spiritual texts
- Following cycles of the moon, astrology, and the seasons
- Supporting political or social causes (through volunteering, donations, or magickal workings)
- Expressing love for others (through words or actions)
- Expressing love for yourself

ANATOMY OF A SELF-CARE RITUAL: COMPONENTS

In addition to the Pillars of Divinity, you'll also want to think about the literal components of your self-care rituals. Especially when you are first starting out with creating your own rituals, it can be very helpful to give the same general structure to all of the rituals that you do, such as starting and ending the same way with each one.

Cleansing is a common way to start off a ritual. In witchcraft, cleansing is the act of purifying your space, body, and mind before engaging in a ritual or magickal working. These are a few popular ways you might incorporate cleansing into your rituals:

- *Smoke cleansing*: Burning cleansing herbs such as sage or cedar and cleansing the air and objects with the resulting smoke.
- *Spray cleansing*: Combine distilled water and essential oils or fresh herbs in a spray bottle and spritz the air with the cleansing combination.
- *Water cleansing*: Literally washing your body and your space with clean water is another way to perform cleansing as part of your ritual.
- *Body scan meditation*: The meditation ritual that you learned in Chapter 2 on page 30 is a great way to mentally cleanse and check in with yourself before a full ritual.

Casting a circle is another way to open your rituals. This is a more traditional form of ritual that is common among Wiccans and official covens and it takes on various forms depending on who you ask. Essentially, a cast circle is a cone of protection that creates sacred space within it. You can perform elaborate rituals to cast a circle including forming a literal circle with salt or chalk, lighting a candle in each of the four cardinal directions, and calling upon the elements to protect you. If you choose to cast a circle, be sure to also close the circle when your ritual is complete.

A formal ending for your rituals can also be very supportive to create a sense of structure. For me, extinguishing the candles I've lit is a very simple but effective method for closing my rituals, but here are a few additional ideas as well:

- *Spoken word*: Simply speak aloud that your ritual is complete.
- *Discard materials*: If you have particular materials you've used during the ritual, such as incense or herbs, mindfully discard them to close your ritual.
- *Yoga and/or meditation*: Move through a particular yoga sequence at the close of each ritual, ending with a meditation or savasana pose.

Tools are also an element of your rituals to consider with care. It's often tempting to incorporate all the tools and techniques and ideas you come across in your studies of witchcraft, but doing so without mindful intention is a recipe for a lifeless and unfulfilling spiritual practice, one you are unlikely to stick with long term. Arbitrarily incorporating spiritual activities into your rituals that might be interesting but don't actually fulfill any particular need of yours is the same as going through the motions of a ritual someone else created, that doesn't speak to any of your own needs.

There are a whole slew of tools that it would appear "most" modern witches use, such as tarot cards, beautifully designed grimoires with regular journaling practices, elaborate altars, and complex astrology charts. But social media, though inspiring, can also be a dark hole of comparison. One of the greatest reasons so many modern witches stray from their path is that they didn't feel they were "doing it right" or that their practice wasn't beautiful enough to be up to their own high standards. Standards that were mostly built on the beautiful but often false view from social media.

This is why it's so important to do the work of allowing your inner child to play and experiment with different tools and ideas so that you can find those that truly work for you. If what you are working with in your witchcraft and self-care practice feels nourishing for you, you'll stop caring if it's Pinterest-worthy. That doesn't mean your practice can't or shouldn't be beautiful; after all, seeking beauty is part of what makes us human. But beauty does not mean something is without flaws, and learning to embrace those flaws is a self-care ritual in and of itself.

Tools are not strictly necessary for your self-care practice at all and it's important to remember that. For one thing, if all of your self-care rituals rely heavily on having access to specific tools, what would you do if you didn't have access to them? Would your entire self-care practice crumble? Sustainability is an important element to think about when choosing the tools you want to work with, if any. That's not to suggest that tools are in any way negative. In fact, working with tools as a witch can help you to powerfully direct your energy and intentions for more effective spells and rituals and the same goes for self-care.

All of these elements, the Five Pillars of Divinity, and the supporting components, can be combined into meaningful and supportive rituals that fulfill your unique self-care needs . . . but how to begin?

CREATING YOUR RITUAL STEP-BY-STEP

As you grow in your self-care practice as a witch, you'll become more and more comfortable creating your own rituals and the creation process will flow through you easily without need for rules. And, in fact, there are no rules in witchcraft which is the beauty of this path! When you're getting started though, it can be helpful to have a certain amount of structure to guide you. You can pretty much mix and match the Five Pillars of Divinity and the closing and ending elements of rituals described above to create your rituals. That's right, it doesn't have to be complicated!

In the first few chapters, you brainstormed spiritual activities that really resonate with you and got additional inspiration from your astrological natal chart. Now we're going to put it all together. There is nothing formulaic about self-care, but creating a formula for yourself that serves your purposes is a great way to start creating rituals with ease. Feel free to adapt the process outlined here in whatever ways best suit you!

Step One: Define Your Purpose

By now you've probably noticed that I always like to begin with journaling. Journaling is just another way of asking your intuition what is right for you, but in a way you can reflect back on later—the perfect combination for self-care! Let's begin with a few questions to get your curiosity piqued about the purpose of a particular ritual and of your self-care and spiritual path in general.

Take the time to get really in tune with your intuition before answering these questions. Maybe go for a walk in nature or do ten minutes of meditation or (yes, I'm going to say it) take a relaxing bubble bath. Doing some intuitive work such as working with your divination tools is also going to help you get deeper with these questions. You may even want to answer the questions and then return to them again tomorrow or on the next full moon to see how your answers can get deeper still.

Why are you pursuing this spiritual path? What enlightenment are you seeking?

_____

_____

_____

What is the root of your need for self-care? What aspects of yourself need the most nourishment?

_____

_____

_____

What change do you want to create in your life with this specific ritual?

_____

_____

_____

When you feel you've identified the purpose of your ritual, start a new page in your self-care grimoire. Write the title of the ritual at the top, if you feel called to give it one. (It can be something simple like "Morning Self-Care Ritual.") Below your title, write down the purpose of the ritual. Don't be afraid to write things down. It does not mean this is set in stone just because it's on paper. What you're doing is creating a record of your growth and experiences. By writing down your rituals as you create them, and then practicing them in the real world, you'll see shifts that need to be made and tweaks that need to happen. Recording that process of evolution is more beautiful than having a pristine grimoire or journal.

One of the frequent challenges I hear from modern witches about their grimoires is that they don't like leaving space to fill in later, because they never know how many lines or how many pages they're going to need, but that they also don't like having all the sections of their grimoires separated. For instance, if you write down the title and purpose and structure (which we'll get to in a moment) of your ritual on page 3 of your grimoire but by the time you want to come back and make notes about the changes you made and why, you're now on page 40, either you need to have left space to make those notes in your original page or your notes will be separated from the ritual itself. Many witches choose to use a binder or scrapbook that you can add pages to as needed so that you can add pages immediately after the ritual, no matter how much of the grimoire you've utilized, and that's one great solution that may work well for you.

Tip: keep it simple by creating a little index at the bottom of each ritual page. You can write something like "See also:" and then fill in with page numbers of related notes as you add to the grimoire. This way you can easily look at that ritual and flip to the relevant pages without needing to save the right amount of space or buy a special binder.

Next, let's explore how to put the pieces of your actual ritual together.

Step Two: Create Your Structure

This is the really fun part. Creating a ritual is very much like baking. The ingredients must be combined in a certain way to achieve the desired effect. Have you ever thought about how most baked goods contain the same basic ingredients like flour, sugar, eggs, milk, and baking powder, yet they can look and taste so vastly different from one another? They can satisfy different cravings depending on how they are combined and in what amounts. The same goes for rituals. Each of the Five Pillars of Divinity are very broad, general categories of the types of "ingredients" you could include in each of your rituals. It may very well be that some of those ingredients are in several or even all of the rituals you perform in your practice. In some rituals, you may focus more on one ingredient than the others or the purpose of an ingredient may differ from how you typically use it.

The Five Pillars of Divinity are essentially a game of mix-and-match. You can engage some or all of them in a ritual and you can highlight any one over the others in a ritual. It's important to get really clear on your purpose before trying to create your structure because as you choose each element, you should be checking it against the purpose of the ritual to see if it fulfills a specific need.

Start by exploring each of the five pillars and how you might engage them in this ritual.

- **Mind:** Will you engage your mental faculties in this ritual? How?

- **Body:** Will you engage your physical experience in this ritual? How?
- **Nature:** Will you engage the power of the natural world in this ritual? How?
- **Divination:** Will you engage with your intuitive wisdom in this ritual? How?
- **Devotional:** Will you engage with the devotion you feel for life in this ritual? How?

Once you've decided which pillars to make use of in this ritual, consider how and why they fulfill your needs. Use the purpose that you've defined as a sort of mission statement. Look objectively at each of the pillar elements you've chosen and ask yourself: Does this serve my mission? How? Why?

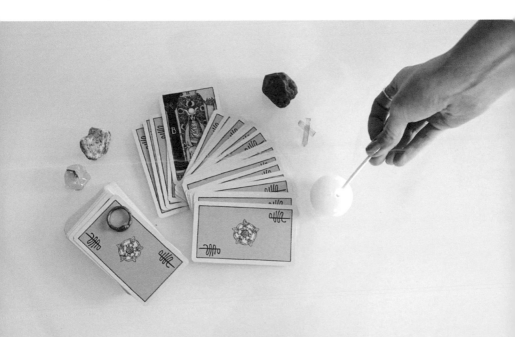

If you come across something you want to include in your ritual that doesn't seem to serve your mission, take the time to get deeper with it. Examine what has drawn you to that element. What about this activity is appealing? Might it be better served in a different ritual or does it not seem to meet your needs at all? There may well be a different side of yourself that needs fulfillment from this element that you haven't considered yet, or there may be something more fulfilling that you can replace that element with to satisfy the same interest or curiosity.

When you've completed these exercises, you should have a clear idea of not only the purpose of this ritual and the needs it will fulfill, but how each of the ingredients works together to fulfill a specific aspect. The ingredients of your ritual should combine in just such a way as to satisfy the particular craving you have set out to fill—just as a pumpkin chocolate chip cookie might satisfy a very different craving than a slice of lemon chiffon cake, even though they probably have many ingredients in common.

First ask yourself which element you will focus on most. This should be governed by the purpose that you've defined for your ritual. For instance, if the purpose is to connect more with your intuition, then perhaps meditation or tarot will be the primary focus, while working with intuitive crystals under the full moon will be supporting players. Each element contributes to the whole but the focus remains on the key aspects. I encourage you to actually rank the importance of each element you've chosen to include, 1 through 5 or however many you have. This will help you understand clearly for yourself what is truly vital to the ritual and what is supportive but less necessary.

Think, too, about how you can combine multiple elements into one single act. For example, I love to choose a crystal related to my ritual, such as a crystal ruled by the moon for moon rituals or a crystal that is associated with the outcome I desire or problem I'm experiencing, and then use that crystal to choose an oracle card when doing a reading. I'll shuffle the deck, fan the cards out in a semi-circle, and then hold the crystal over the cards until I feel drawn to one. This combines a divination element of reading cards, a body element of holding crystals, and even a nature element of working with the raw energy of the crystal itself. All in one go! Creative combinations of elements like this can help make your rituals more concise without sacrificing all the things you want to include.

Step Three: Choosing Your Tools & Supporting Components
Last, you'll put the finishing touches on your ritual by choosing your tools and other components. Think very practically for a moment about the ingredients and activities you've chosen to structure your ritual around. Jot down a list of all the "things" you need to perform them.

If you're working with divination tools, then, of course, you'll need your tools, like your tarot cards or your pendulum. If you're doing any kind of journaling, you need a journal and a pen. If you plan to take ritual baths, you'll need, well, a bathtub, and any herbs or crystals you'll be including. Answer these questions and allow yourself to get curious about the possibilities of working with or without tools:

- What physical or imaginary tools will you use in this ritual? What supplies do you need?
- If you had to perform this ritual without any tools, would it be possible?

Note any of the things on your list that you don't actually have yet. Consider this a bit like a shopping list of what you need to perform the ritual exactly as you've envisioned, but remember that tools are never *necessary* for witchcraft or self-care. With that in mind, you may want to ask yourself if you can adapt the rituals to be tool-free or if these additional acquisitions are worthwhile for you.

If there is anything that is impossible or impractical for you to acquire right now, think about how you can adapt the ritual to still fulfill the need without feeling like you're making a sacrifice. Take the bathtub example: if you don't live somewhere that actually has a bathtub, consider making the ritual into a foot bath or a hand soak instead. There is always a creative solution that can find the balance between your reality and your ideal.

Finally, consider the opening, closing, and cleansing portions of your ritual. These are not mandatory but they do help give your ritual a sense of form. What type of cleansing will you perform in this ritual? It may be that you wish to use the same type of cleansing for all of your rituals for consistency, but you can also mix it up. As we talked about at the beginning of this chapter, consistency and repetition are commonly thought of as part of the definition of ritual, and whether those are concepts you value is up to you. Personally, I use a variety of cleansing tools depending on my mood and what I feel most called to use. Some days I burn incense, some days I diffuse cleansing essential oils, and some days I use a cleansing spray like Florida water. There are many options and you may well wish to experiment with them all, as each has its own tone and personality, so your needs may vary depending on the ritual you are performing.

Opening and closing your ritual are perhaps the most formal

parts of any ritual as you need something to focus your mind at the beginning and to release all the work you've done at the end. Think about how you will formally (or informally, with intention) begin and end your ritual. The level of formality with which you open and close your ritual sort of sets the tone, so consider the mood you want to be in for your ritual. What kind of feeling do you want to invoke during and after?

All of these elements, from cleansing and casting circles to divination and meditation and ritual bathing and all the other things you could include in your self-care rituals, represent your unique spiritual worldview. The things you consider important, the tools you desire to work with, and the way that you engage with the Five Pillars of Divinity are all calling to you for a reason. They are messages from your higher self or the divine or the spirit realm, wherever you receive messages from that are meant for your deepest, truest self. Your self-care experience is your own and all you need do to create meaningful rituals is follow your intuition and your heart to whatever is calling to you.

Follow those bread crumbs!

Chapter 5
START & END THE DAY WITH SELF-CARE

Now that you have more of a clear picture of what is motivating you to embrace a self-care practice and of generally how to put together your own rituals, we can start creating real-world rituals, not only hypothetical ones! In the third part of this book, you'll find suggested self-care rituals of all kinds to activate your mind, body, intuition, connection to nature, and sense of devotion. You might be wondering why we aren't starting there: wouldn't it be easier to create rituals once you've seen a bunch of ideas of how rituals can fit together?

Perhaps, but I've laid out this book in a particular order with a lot of intention. Although sometimes it is easier to get inspiration from others when creating your spiritual practice, I find it results in a more fulfilling result if you ask your intuition what you should do *first* and look for inspiration from outside of yourself second. There is definitely nothing wrong with gathering inspiration from a variety of sources, taking all the best parts of an existing idea, and combining those with your own thoughts. But it's important to remember that you actually do have all the tools you need inside of you, especially when it comes to creating a spiritual practice that is fulfilling of your own unique needs. That's why taking the time to ask your intuition what kind of rituals are going to light you up and nourish you in all the best ways *before* seeking additional inspiration is the most powerful action you can take.

To begin with, we're going to create morning and evening self-care rituals that suit your own unique lifestyle, schedule, beliefs, and the needs that you have identified. When working with my spiritual coaching clients, I always like to start with morning and evening rituals because this is such a great, approachable place to begin. You already have morning and evening rituals whether you even realize it or not: brushing your teeth, packing a lunch, bathing routines, reading before bed, these are all rituals. They might seem terribly mundane but each of these mini-acts that you perform every day is part of your overall self-care practice. After all, self-care begins with the basics of caring for your physical needs like health and hygiene.

But how can you go about making these seemingly mundane, boring, and necessary activities into part of a fulfilling spiritual practice as a witch?

The trick is to incorporate a little bit of magick and a little bit of mundane into all parts of your morning and evening routines and to draw the spiritual side of these practices into your daily life in a sustainable way. When you first begin practicing as a witch, it's tempting to want to do magick 24–7. Whenever you're doing mundane necessities, you feel like they are all the more boring and whenever you don't have time to do all of the many magickal activities you're interested in over the course of a busy day (or week, or month), you feel like a "bad witch." The reality is that you can't do magick all the time, nor can you expect to experience spiritual connection if you're always focused on your mundane responsibilities, nor can you expect to be able to fit everything you want to do into the same twenty-four hours that you've always had, without making some adjustments. You need to balance all aspects of yourself in order to truly care for yourself as a whole.

We've all been in that space where it just feels like you're the worst witch, because you never seem to have time for your practice. I'm not a morning person at all, and given the opportunity, I'll sleep in until 8:00 or 9:00 a.m. every day (or later on a lazy Sunday morning, as my boyfriend will tell you). When I was working a regular nine-to-five day job, before I quit to pursue my dreams of being a spiritual coach and professional witch, I would typically roll out of bed twenty- to thirty-five minutes before I had to leave for work. All I had time to do in the mornings was the bare necessities: brush my teeth and hair, throw on makeup and clothes, and *maybe* toss a bagel in the toaster that I would scarf down in the car. There was certainly no making the bed, no yoga flow, no mindfully chosen cup of tea, none of the things that I daydreamed about doing as part of a nourishing morning ritual.

Tea rituals are a big part of my spiritual practice. Giving my attention to the process of making a cup of tea and taking that first sip is deeply fulfilling for me. And yet at that time in my life, I was drinking my first cup of tea from a to-go mug at my desk or in my first meeting of the day. I would suck down at least six to eight more cups throughout the work day without thinking about the mindful process of steeping and sipping that is otherwise so important to me. I tried again and again to find ways to force myself to get up earlier so that I could have this magical, fairy-tale morning ritual that I had dreamed of. Nothing worked. Gentle alarm clocks that woke me up as I emerged from REM sleep. Meditation alarm clocks that woke me up with a yoga sequence in bed. Every new thing I tried would work for a few days or a few weeks and I would get all excited that I was going to start getting up earlier, but then eventually I would be right back where I had started.

It's not as if I wasn't productive during the day; my inner Virgo rising is all about productivity! But I'm not productive first thing in the morning and that's okay. Over time, I developed a morning ritual that was slightly more bespoke to my needs but still honored the fact that I just couldn't get myself up any earlier than I already was, a fact I had to accept about myself. In the last few months that I worked a regular nine-to-five job, I would go downstairs and turn the kettle on before I brushed my teeth so that the water was hot for my tea by the time I was finished. Then I'd light a few candles and pull an oracle card at my vanity before doing my makeup, all while sipping a cup of tea. If I really felt motivated, I might do a few sun salutations. It really was working and although I still didn't feel like I had time to make the bed or eat breakfast at home, at least I was doing something. I had felt like something of a fraud for always talking to my clients about how fulfilling having a morning ritual can be but not really having a satisfying one of my own so I was immensely grateful for this feeling of accomplishment.

And then the universe threw a wrench into my new routines. As I described in Chapter 2 on page 26, I became incredibly and mysteriously sick with a terrible reaction to . . . something. I was on Prednisone for three solid weeks and barely slept for almost a month. Eventually, I felt like myself again and could go back to work, but I was never officially diagnosed with anything in particular.

Those few weeks of illness, followed by leaving my day job just a few short weeks after that, took me out of my routines completely. My morning ritual was, frankly, shot.

But here's the thing: once I was working for myself and could set my own schedule, all of a sudden, I started making my bed every day. This little, mundane thing that I had felt guilty my entire adult life about not doing, suddenly became part of my average day. It was like a switch had flipped.

I'll be honest, I'm still negotiating with myself about what my morning ritual is supposed to look like, but I can say from experience that your daily rituals are not a static thing. You do not create them once and then "set it and forget it," so to speak. Your daily rituals and all parts of your spiritual practice are an ever-evolving experience that you have to be willing and able to flow with. All of that is to say I guarantee that the morning and evening ritual you create through the work you'll do in this chapter will not be the exact morning and evening rituals you'll be practicing a year from now. However, doing this work to understand what it is that's nourishing for you and to accept that you will feel varying levels of commitment and motivation for your daily practice at different times in your life, is going to set you up for all kinds of fulfillment.

MORNING RITUALS

Mornings are often described as the most important part of your day because how you start off the day is how you will carry yourself through the rest of it. If you're not a morning person, like me, that

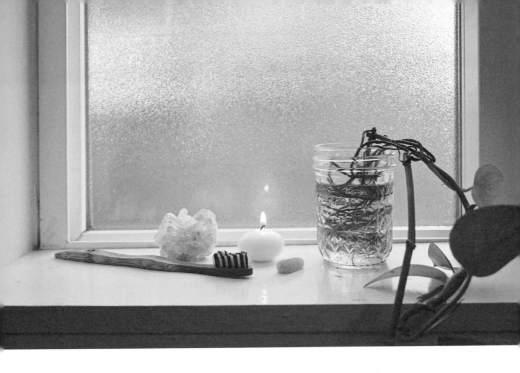

might make you groan and wonder how early you have to start getting up *now*, just so you can squeeze a little ritual in. But that's not the idea here: your morning ritual shouldn't feel like it's something you have to drag yourself out of bed for nor should it be something you just go through the motions of while you're still half asleep!

Your rituals are not something to be shoehorned into your life. If you're not a morning person, then maybe a morning ritual just isn't for you.

Shocked to hear that in a chapter about morning and evening rituals?

Well, I'm not here to tell you that 5:00 a.m. is a mystical and dreamy time of day when all of your biggest intentions and dreams can be manifested and that if you don't get up until 9:00 a.m., you're never going to manifest much of anything or that sleeping in is somehow contrary to self-care.

I'm also not ever here to tell you what your rituals or your spiritual practice is supposed to look like.

But if creating a morning ritual feels like it is self-care and it is something you want to experience (because your intuition said so, not because I said so or because anyone else said so), then let's explore the tools to make it happen.

Your morning self-care ritual in particular is always going to be a combination of the magickal and the mundane, simply because we all lead busy lives and we have things to do in the mornings. That's why it's so important to take into account what you need to accomplish in the morning besides spiritual connection and how much time you realistically have.

FIGURING OUT WHAT YOUR MORNING RITUAL NEEDS TO DO FOR YOU

Tomorrow morning, I recommend you do the following exercise so you can get an idea of the kinds of activities that are essential to your morning:

Before you go to bed tonight, lay out a piece of paper and a pen beside your bed. When you wake up, write down what time it is and note whether you are up early, late, or on time, and by how much.

Move through all of the daily, mundane activities that you always do, such as brushing your teeth, getting dressed, etc. As you start each new activity, turn on the timer on your smartphone and then record on the paper how long each activity takes. Your paper should look something like this:

Woke up: 6:22 a.m. (7 minutes late)

Brushed teeth: 4 minutes

Styled hair: 11 minutes

Applied makeup: 13 minutes

Got dressed: 6 minutes

Cooked breakfast: 17 minutes

Packed lunch for the kids: 14 minutes

When you next work on creating your morning ritual, pull out this record and look it over carefully. Is there anything that surprises you? Any activity that takes way longer than it seems like it should or anything that you always thought was taking up a ton of your time in the morning that's actually pretty short? Is there anything you could do the night before to save yourself time in the morning?

Now, make a list of all the magickal self-care activities you *wish* you could incorporate into your ideal morning, if you had all the time and privacy in the world. Really allow yourself to brain dump here and don't hold anything back because it seems unrealistic. No self-limitation: this is the time for being unrealistic and allowing yourself to dream! You can ask yourself the following questions as inspiration:

- What time would you get up each day if you had no other specific obligations? Would it be earlier or later than you currently get up?
- In what ways does your current morning ritual feel fulfilling?
- Which aspects of yourself do not feel nourished by your current morning ritual (mental or physical health, emotional self, intuition, astrological self-care needs, etc.)?

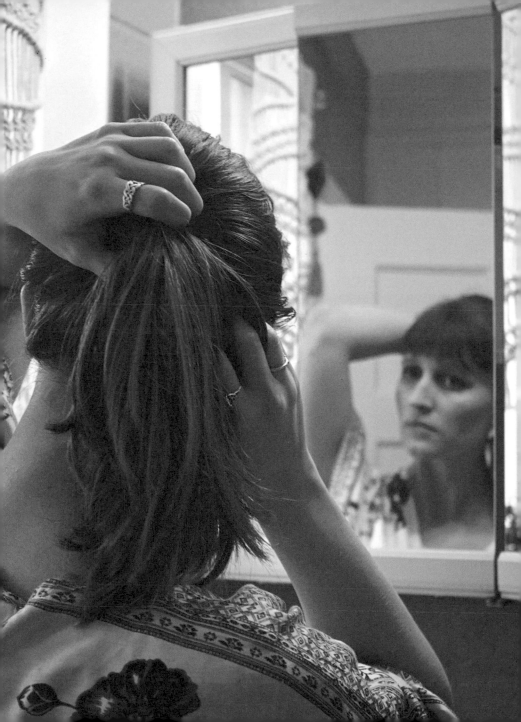

- Are there any aspects of your morning routine that feel stressful or frustrating?

When you've completed these exercises, you should be able to think about your current morning routine in terms of what is possible. You've thought about what your morning self-care ritual could look like without any other obligations or restrictions on your time.

Now, think about how you can create a magickal, self-care-focused morning that *honors* the restrictions on your time, because self-care is not about avoiding responsibilities or trying to force space into your busy day for huge chunks of indulgent, self-care activities. Self-care is about finding ways to care for yourself *within the boundaries of your actual lifestyle.* Trying to create elaborate self-care rituals that you don't actually have time for is only going to become an additional source of stress, defeating the whole purpose in the first place!

So, what does that look like in your real life? It might mean rearranging your morning schedule so that you do have more time. But it may also look like finding ways to practice magick and self-care while doing mundane activities.

Don't think brushing your teeth can be witchy? Think again! Here are a few examples of how you can turn even the most mundane activities into magickal self-care:

- Brushing your teeth: Create a mantra that you can repeat in your head a certain number of times while brushing your teeth. The repetitive motion will focus your mind and boost the energy of the mantra and you can use it to time how long you've been brushing for, too!

- Applying makeup: Witches often like to use makeup as a glamour, a spell that makes other people see you a certain way. As you're applying your makeup, infuse the act with the intention to highlight your inner beauty and light.
- Making coffee: Stir cream or sugar into your coffee in a clockwise (*deosil*) motion to invite in good things or in a counterclockwise (*widdershins*) motion to banish negativity from your day.

As you can see, just about any activity can be made into a moment of magick in your morning. Look back over your timeline that you created to track your morning routine. Which of those activities that you are already doing could become more magickal? More importantly, which ones would feel more nourishing if you introduced an element of magick?

I don't recommend trying to incorporate magick into every single thing you do, though, at least not at first. Think mindfully about your own needs as you've identified them and create an element of your morning ritual to address each specific need. If there's a magickal activity you want to experiment with that doesn't meet a particular need, ask yourself why you're drawn to it: maybe that activity would fulfill a need you hadn't even realized you had yet. Always return to the anatomy of a self-care ritual that you learned in the last chapter. Although it's tempting to think that the purpose of a morning or evening ritual is to start or end your day with self-care, that's really just a side benefit. Identifying the deeper purpose of your self-care ritual first will give you a strong foundation to build on instead of arbitrarily trying to bolt various magickal activities onto your current mundane routines without reason.

Keep in mind that it can be all too easy to fall into the trap of negative self-talk when your ideal magickal morning self-care ritual doesn't measure up to reality. Like I said, your morning ritual is going to evolve with your needs and, perhaps most importantly, with your schedule. Sometimes, you have more time and more motivation than other times. Schedules change with the seasons and can be dependent on work, school, and hobbies. It's not just the things you're *obligated* to do that can keep you from your self-care and spiritual practice, sometimes it's the thing you're excited to do too, and there just isn't enough time in the day.

If right now your morning routine looks something like my harried, thirty-minute situation once did, that's perfectly okay. There is always room for growth and improvement and it's entirely acceptable to not always have it all together.

Perhaps the first rule of self-care is accepting yourself exactly as you are, and this applies to all aspects of your life. I really invite you to embrace the journey toward self-acceptance. The second rule of self-care, though, is that making self-care a priority is the only way it's going to become an integral part of your rituals and routines. So, crafting a morning self-care ritual that feels good and nourishing and doesn't make you feel guilty for not doing more is about striking the balance between what you truly have time for and what is sustainable versus also making sure that you're treating self-care like a priority in your life.

EVENING RITUALS

Evening rituals are a very different beast than morning rituals. In some ways, there's more room for magick in an evening ritual as it's likely that you have fewer mundane obligations at night, though that could vary greatly depending on your lifestyle and schedule. In broad terms, though, evening rituals can really fulfill your need for rest and relaxation or for deeper, spiritual connection—or perhaps even do both at the same time!

They say midnight is the "witching hour" for a reason; nighttime is when you tap into your deepest self, your darkest or most taboo needs, and learn to really embrace your inner witch. Many people like to perform rituals under the light of the moon, and this is the time of romantic trysts and erotic interludes as well. Nighttime is also when you sleep, of course, when you tap into the dream realm. As you learned in Chapter 2 on page 34, dreams are the gateway to your intuition which is what makes dream journaling so powerful. The lunar cycle can have a huge impact on your emotions and your intuitive power too and watching the moon rise is a powerful way to get in touch with those cycles.

As you can see, there is lots of room for integrating your spiritual practice into an evening self-care ritual. You might consider incorporating certain "mundane" elements into your evening ritual, such as brushing your teeth, washing your face, applying moisturizer, or "unplugging" and setting aside all electronics an hour before bed, but even these take on a more magickal element in the evening. Your hygiene routines can become more indulgent as you prepare for bed than when you're getting ready for the day. The process of

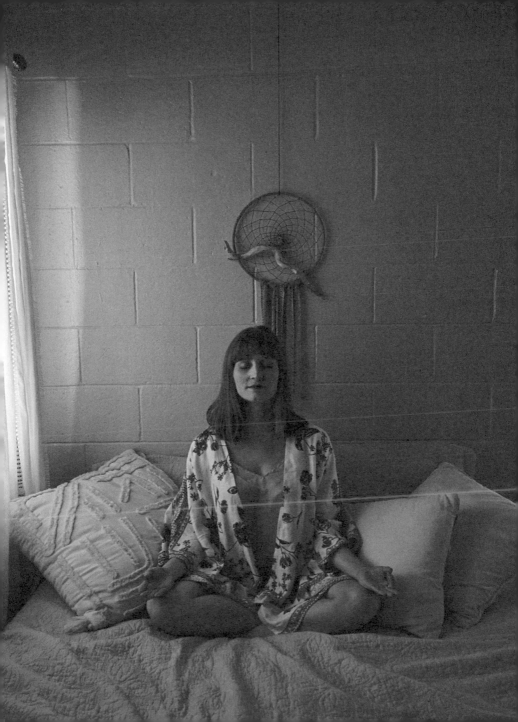

disconnecting from the technological stress of the day can become one of connecting with the mindful peace of true solitude.

The biggest challenge with creating nourishing evening rituals is often that we don't have as much of a solid foundation to work from. In the morning, there are almost always certain routines that you pretty much do every day and even if they feel entirely mundane, as you learned, there are lots of ways to incorporate magick into them. In the evening though, it's very easy to slip into non-routine routines, where you're doing things like watching TV at night or hanging out with friends instead of having a solid nightly ritual.

If that's the case for you, no need to feel bad. It's always a good idea to go about creating a new ritual with your eyes wide open so that you not only recognize the individual needs that the ritual should fulfill but also so that you're aware of the potential challenges. If you aren't accustomed to devoting time in the evening to your spiritual and self-care practice, you might experience a period of growing pains while you sort out exactly what's going to work for you.

This is where we return to the anatomy of a self-care ritual and, first, define the purpose of your evening practice. As you start to think about what you want your evening ritual to look like, ask yourself if you're looking for a more restorative experience or if you want to use this time to deepen your connection to your intuition or to the divine.

Restorative experiences might suit you better if you are often very tired at the end of the day, if you spend a lot of time serving others in one way or another (everyone from service workers to parents might fall here), or if you suffer from chronic pain or illness, significant stress, or depression. Restoration can focus on restoring your spirit, restoring your desire to give generously, restoring your faith, or restoring your unstressed mind and body.

Deepening your connection to your spirituality might be a better fit for your evening rituals if you're more of a night person and have more energy to put into it. If study, research, and reading feel exciting and nourishing to you, then your evening ritual is the perfect opportunity to make a little time in your day for those activities. It's also the perfect time for practicing your craft as a witch and exploring what that means to you, especially if you can eke out some alone time in the evenings for intuitive readings and spell work.

The thing is, "restorative" and "connective" can mean very different things to different people. You need to figure out what they mean to you and how you might fulfill those needs with your evening self-care practice, as we all really need a balance of both, regardless of which you focus on more. Evening is the time of day when we take a step back from our busy lives and set aside the masks we wear the rest of the time. Whoever you are underneath the masks you wear (the masks of partner, colleague, parent, friend, etc.), that person is at least an aspect of your inner witch, as your inner witch is the deepest, truest part of yourself.

In what ways does your inner witch need restoration? Where does she feel malnourished and neglected? In what ways do you feel particularly exhausted, stressed, or frustrated? What would it feel like if you could let go of those feelings? In what ways does your inner witch crave deeper connection? Where does she feel out of touch and out of sync with her true purpose? How have you been hiding from opportunities for deeper connection? In following the pattern

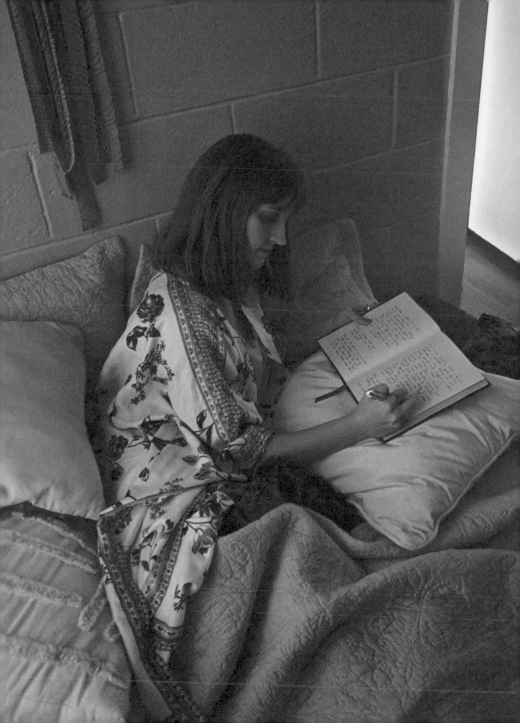

that you learned in Chapter 4 on page 93, once you've identified the purpose of your ritual, it's time to figure out the structure.

Restorative self-care practices include activities like ritual bathing, yin yoga, bedtime meditation, and self-massage. Activities that will help you deepen your spiritual connection could include nightly tarot readings or other divination practices, learning and researching about spiritual topics that interest you, and working with your chakras. The beauty of an evening ritual is that, depending on your own interests and needs, you can incorporate a variety of restorative and connective activities!

Evening rituals are the perfect time for one of my favorite self-care tools: self-reflection. The ability to reflect on your own actions, thoughts, and feelings is one of the things that makes you uniquely human and which connects you to your highest self and to the divine. Self-reflection can be a very restorative experience or can help you get really deep and intimate with yourself, so finding which variation works for you will be important, as will allowing yourself to flow and evolve with the practice over time.

Journaling on one of the many prompts and questions in this book is a great place to get started with self-reflection. Recording your thoughts on paper in your own handwriting is known to be a powerful way to process emotions and trauma, transmute shadows, break down internal barriers, and bring new ideas into reality. I think this is because the power of self-reflection is unlimited. When you take the time to stop and think about your own thoughts, words, actions, and feelings, you are stepping into alignment with the divine, whatever that means to you. This is something that only gods and humans are really capable of doing and it's your birthright to get deep with yourself in this way.

Ask yourself where you feel a lack of depth and intimacy in your life. Where do you feel like you don't fully understand your own motivations? Astrologically speaking, the signs and houses that Venus and Scorpio show up within your chart will be very insightful for your relationship with these concepts of intimacy and depth. Allow yourself to get curious about these aspects of yourself and take the time each evening to get more in touch with them.

Your evening self-care ritual is an opportunity to invite intimacy into your spiritual practice. When you've taken the time to really do this inner work, get in touch with your inner witch and embrace the needs that are unique to you. Creating a restorative and nourishing ritual will be an exercise in intimacy with yourself. After all, self-care is not a surface-level experience, and you have to get deep beneath your own layers to discover how to create fulfillment from within.

WHY STARTING AND ENDING THE DAY WITH SELF-CARE IS SO POWERFUL

Morning and evening rituals are certainly an easy way to get started on creating your own self-care rituals. They're easy to conceptualize because you probably already have some kind of morning and evening routine to build off of. That's not the only reason these are the first rituals I recommend you create though; morning and evening rituals are important in and of themselves. They give you an opportunity to start and end the day with self-care. Morning and evening rituals bookend your day with positivity. The way that you begin and end the day sticks with you. The way you wake up and the way you fall asleep. These are the moments that program your attitude and your ability to see beyond the present. When you prioritize your*self* in those first and last moments of the day, you are training your brain to see those times as sacred.

Your self-care practice is not something you simply sneak in whenever you have a spare minute. Your self-care practice is a time for sacred devotion to you. Imagine the power, then, of expressing sacred devotion to yourself at the beginning and end of each and every day. Imagine what you can reach and achieve when your mornings and evenings are an expression of your deepest beliefs and an opportunity for growth. But, don't get me wrong, sometimes a morning of sleeping in and cinnamon rolls for breakfast at 11:00 am or an evening of binging Netflix and falling asleep by the light of the TV is exactly what you need. Rituals can take on many forms . . .

Chapter 6
ADAPT YOUR RITUALS FOR SUSTAINABILITY

Rituals are a big part of the path of the witch. We perform rituals for all aspects of our spirituality, though they can look quite different from witch to witch. There are moon rituals, seasonal sabbat rituals, private rituals, group rituals, structured religious rituals, and free-flowing personal rituals.

Rituals can take the form of self-care specifically, such as bathing rituals and meditation, but all rituals can be a form of self-care as well. Rituals give you an opportunity to reconnect with yourself, with your intuition, and with a higher power (whether that's a god, nature, or just your higher self). It's so easy to fall into the trap of feeling like a "bad witch" when you aren't practicing regularly, even though there are so many ways you can be pulled out of your habits.

Everything from vacation to illness to schedule and season changes to depression can disrupt your good habits and keep you from practicing your spirituality or any other forms of self-care. It's all-important to be gentle with yourself when this happens. Mentally berating yourself is not going to get you anywhere and it's actually only going to take you deeper into a place where you don't feel it's worth it to practice at all.

I often hear from the perfectionist Virgo types (of which I definitely am one) that if they can't do their full ritual in exactly the way they planned, they get discouraged, throw their hands up, and figure they might as well not do anything at all. Or I'll hear from my beauty oriented Librans that if their altar or spiritual space isn't set up perfectly, they get distracted and . . . also throw their hands up and figure they might as well not do anything at all. Every sign and every witch has a reason to get discouraged and throw their hands up in frustration.

Luckily, there are many ways to adapt your rituals to make them more sustainable, more anxiety proof, and more able to actually do their job. Because when your rituals are susceptible to mundane assaults like changes in schedule or illness, they are that much less likely to withstand internal attacks like anxiety, fear, and self-doubt. This is especially important for those with chronic pain or illness, those who are caregivers for children with special needs, anyone whose life can be interrupted at any moment by the needs of their body or those around them.

Creating rituals that are adaptable and built to actually fit into your life, instead of trying to force your reality into the confines of a ritual you've created, is absolutely essential to a spiritual self-care practice that you can realistically maintain.

LEAVING SPACE FOR THE REALITIES OF LIFE

I find it helpful, especially when you are just getting started, to create a few different variations of your daily rituals, so that when life gets in the way, you aren't thrown for a total loop. When illness, work, family, or vacation keeps you from being able to practice every day in the way you've envisioned, instead of getting discouraged, you can turn to one of the ritual variations you've created!

By creating these different variations of your ideal rituals, you don't have to sacrifice the whole thing when you don't have time or motivation. Often, when we can't practice in exactly the way we envisioned, we throw the metaphorical baby out with the ritual bathwater and choose not to practice at all. It's sort of a throw-your-hands-in-the-air scenario, where if it can't be perfect then what's the point? But when you toss your rituals aside because they aren't perfect, they're doing you even less good than when you carry on with beautiful imperfection. Next time you wake up late or have a fun party to go to in the evening, don't just throw your hands in the air and give up on the spiritual self-care rituals you've created. Instead, turn to one of the variations you've developed with intention for just this situation. It's empowering to already have a plan in place for those unexpected times when your typical practice just isn't possible. Instead of feeling dejected and like a "bad witch" for abandoning your rituals, you get to feel bolstered by knowing just what to do to support your own needs in any situation.

Here's an example of how this can work:

Your Primary Ritual: This is the full ritual you've created for an ideal situation.

Your Abbreviated Ritual: This is an abbreviated version of your ritual, in which you might remove or shorten some of the lengthier aspects of the ritual to save time. For example, if you usually do a three-card tarot reading in the morning, you could pull just one card, or you could skip the reading altogether. Especially in the case of morning rituals, whichever aspect of your ritual you remove, just make sure it's not something that's going to leave you feeling unfinished throughout the day. You'll find that some elements of your ritual feel more important than others so try not to remove the essentials unless absolutely necessary.

Your Mini-Ritual: This is about breaking your primary ritual down into a bunch of little bite-sized chunks, so on those crazy mornings when you've overslept, you can pick and choose just one or two mini-rituals to help you feel connected and nourished, even when you don't have time for a full ritual at all.

MINI-RITUALS

Whatever struggle or shadow is keeping you from practicing self-care and your spirituality, mini-rituals are at least part of the solution. Mini-rituals are all the little activities and tasks that make up your larger rituals, but that you can perform on their own for a similar impact. Every ritual is made up of many parts, so in this chapter, we're going to look at how you can break up your daily rituals and also how you can do this with larger rituals like those you might perform for the sabbats or moon phases and why this is an act of self-care in and of itself.

Mini-rituals are actually kind of a way to trick your conscious mind, the part of you that can be hyper self-critical and the voice in your head that says if it's not perfect, it's worthless. We all go through experiences and times in our life when the perfect ideal is just not going to be reality. Mini-rituals can be a wonderful, supportive device to employ during those times.

I discovered mini-rituals when I was navigating the process of creating my own fulfilling morning self-care ritual, as I described in the last chapter. This has been something of an ongoing process for much of my life, as I'm just not a morning person! For me, being a witch is my self-care practice. I won't bore you with *all* the astrological details but suffice it to say that I have a stellium in the eighth house and I'm part of the Pluto in Scorpio generation so witchcraft is a driving force in my life. At a time when I was struggling most to have any kind of morning practice, or even any kind of magickal practice at all, mini-rituals came along and revealed themselves to me just when I needed them most.

I was trying in vain one morning to get a little bit of spiritual practice in before I had to go to work and struck a match to light

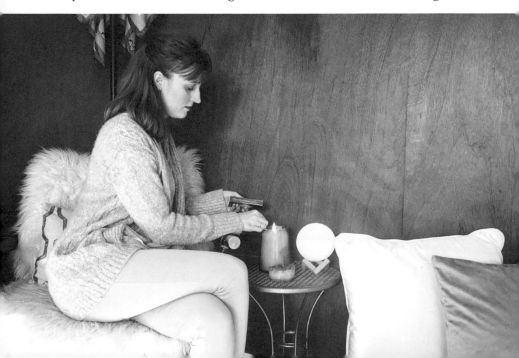

some candles on my altar. I figured that was about as far as I was going to get but at least it would be something.

I struck the match, watched the flame flare at the end of it, and felt myself relax a bit, felt my mind clear. I touched the flame to the candle wick, watched it catch fire, then lifted the match and carefully blew it out. I watched the candle flame dance for a moment and felt some of my stress melt away.

Then it struck me: I had just performed a ritual. Lighting candles was not just the precursor to every ritual I had ever done . . . it was a ritual in and of itself.

This simple thought was a complete and utter revelation and it, honestly, revolutionized the way that I thought about my spiritual and self-care practice. Lighting a candle each morning while I do my makeup is an essential part of starting my day—and it's not just a slacker way of pretending I did a ritual, it is a ritual.

Yes, certainly, I do longer rituals too, especially on the new and full moons and on the pagan sabbats. But lighting a candle each day, feeling the power of fire held between my fingertips in the form of a match, watching the wick flare with flame and then flicker, dancing, warming my face . . . that is all the ritual I really need to feel guided toward connection with my spirituality.

You can break any ritual down into a multitude of parts. In fact, I guarantee that even if you think you've broken your rituals down into their smallest possible parts, you can go just a little bit further, make them just a little bit more, well, mini.

The tea ritual is a great example of how you can break any ritual down into mini-rituals. Its purpose in expressing your spirituality and practicing self-care could vary greatly. But the tea ritual is in fact a series of small acts, each of which represent the Five Pillars of Divinity and the elements individually. First, you pick the plants from the ground or select a tea made from particular plants (nature–Earth). Then, you heat the water and pour it over the prepared tea (nature–fire). Next, you watch as the tea steeps and meditate on its slow curls of color (mind). Then, you lift the teacup to your lips and take a sip (body). Finally, perhaps, you pour additional cups of tea and share them with others or read the leaves (divination or devotion).

In the case of the tea ritual, you can't really perform the final steps of sipping and sharing the tea without first preparing the leaves, heating the water, and steeping the tea blend, but you can choose to give more focus to certain aspects of the full ritual over others. For example, you could give most of your attention to selecting the herbs to brew your tea with, then allow the water to heat and the tea to steep while doing other things. Or, you could choose an easy bagged tea and let it steep while focused on other activities, then give the bulk of your attention to the act of actually consuming the brewed tea.

To offer another example of the anatomy of a self-care ritual, let's look at a daily tarot or oracle card reading. Daily readings are a great way to connect with your intuition and learn to trust the signs it gives you. This is a great example because a tarot reading can be as simple or as involved as you would like it to be.

Here is one potential ritual you could perform around a tarot reading:

First, intuitively select the deck you want to use. Cleanse the deck by waving sage or cedar smoke around it or by sprinkling a ring of sea salt on your altar around the deck (cleansing). Then, choose a

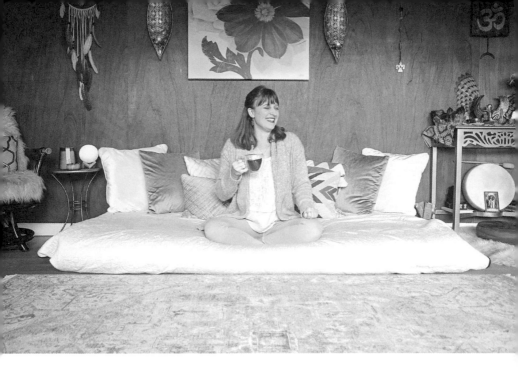

crystal to select your cards. Shuffle the deck and lay the cards out, face down, in a half circle in front of you. Holding the crystal in your hands, move it a few inches above the cards until you feel drawn to choose a particular card (body & divination). Draw the card you've chosen out of the deck and lay it face up on your altar. Consider the symbolism of the card and journal about whatever it intuitively brings up for you (mind & divination).

In this example ritual, you have engaged in quite a few different steps, from selecting a deck and cleansing it to using an outside tool to choose a card and finally journaling about the card you've chosen. When, in fact, you could perform this ritual without several of these pieces, including cleansing, utilizing the crystal, or even journaling about it.

This is where mini-rituals come in. Sometimes, you just don't have time for the full ritual. Perhaps this involved practice of smoke cleansing, healing crystals, and journaling is part of your ideal daily divination ritual, but on certain mornings of the week, during certain times of the year, or due to illness or vacation, you just don't have time for all of this.

By setting up mini-rituals as acceptable alternatives to begin with, you're giving yourself permission to perform a specific part of your ritual, even though you aren't doing the whole thing. Perhaps you would just shuffle your deck, select a card, and meditate on it for a few minutes. Or perhaps your mini-ritual is somewhere in between: you could shuffle the deck, use a crystal to select a card, and then meditate on it, or shuffle the deck, pick a card, and do your journaling.

I recommend that mini-rituals take no longer than five minutes and involve no more than three components, though there are no set rules as to what these should look like and you should always follow your intuition first. I encourage you to write out all of your ideal rituals and then try to break them down into the smallest actions you possibly can. Even if you never perform some of the smallest rituals you come up with, it really is powerful to understand the fundamental building blocks of your practice.

YOUR NATURAL RHYTHMS

I find that one of the most common things that interrupts my clients' spiritual and self-care practices is the changing of the seasons. Though it seems like such a simple thing that many of us experience many times over the course of a lifetime, it's not always a simple obstacle to overcome. I believe this is because we take the seasons for granted and don't live in tune with their rhythms, nor are we in sync with our natural rhythms either.

Our natural rhythms are not necessarily the same as the literal seasonal rhythms. Just as we are all affected by what's happening in the stars generally (like how your computer always seems to go haywire during Mercury Retrograde), but the astrological transits affect you in unique ways depending on your own natal chart, the seasons all affect us in general, collective ways but you have your own relationship with each season as well.

Understanding how the seasons affect you personally is a proactive way to allow your rituals some breathing room to evolve and adapt with the seasonal changes. In general, I find that summer is often a hard time for people to stick with their rituals and self-care practices because they get busy and distracted with all the fun of summer and even just the longer daylight hours. In fall and winter, many people are ready to retreat and turn within so self-care becomes a focus again.

Even just an awareness of these social and seasonal ebbs and flows will give you the tools to prepare yourself for them. You can incorporate more mini-rituals into your life in the spring and summer and make nature walks and spending time out in the sunshine part of your regular practice, for example. You can get so much deeper with this though and, in fact, you can turn again to your astrological natal chart for help in understanding your own natural rhythms. As you learned in Chapter 3 on page 48, your ascendant sign is the constellation that was rising over the eastern horizon at the moment of your birth. You'll need to know your exact birth time in order to calculate the ascendant but if you do have that information available, it's a powerful source of wisdom in your chart.

The ascendant sign is always the sign of the first house and so it determines the signs of all twelve houses in your chart. Because each of the seasons naturally occurs at the cusp of a particular house, each season falls at a particular point in your chart, and you can follow the sun around your chart throughout the year. The natural placement of the seasons on the astrological chart is:

- Spring begins on the first day of Aries season, on the cusp of the first house
- Summer begins on the first day of Cancer season, on the cusp of the fourth house
- Fall begins on the first day of Libra season, on the cusp of the seventh house
- Winter begins on the first day of Capricorn season, on the cusp of the tenth house

Depending on your ascendant sign, you may have different signs in each of these four important houses. One way to implement this information in your life is to follow the sun around your own chart and see where you may experience the energies of the seasons at incongruent times of the year. For example, my ascendant is in Virgo and so I could say that I experience the energies of spring on the cusp of my first house, beginning in late August. For me, it's the excitement and anticipation of back to school season . . . even though I've been out of school for many years now. Each of the ascendant signs experiences the seasons a bit differently and understanding the natural rhythms of the sun as it moves around your chart throughout the year is one way to prepare to adapt your rituals in advance of those rhythmic shifts instead of being blindsided by them.

The following summarizes when during the year each ascendant sign may experience their period of highest energy and of retreat:

- **Aries Rising:** Highest energy at the spring equinox, begins to retreat and turn inward at the autumn equinox
- **Taurus Rising:** Highest energy in late spring, begins to retreat and turn inward in late autumn
- **Gemini Rising:** Highest energy in early summer, begins to retreat and turn inward in early winter
- **Cancer Rising:** Highest energy at the summer solstice, begins to retreat and turn inward at the winter solstice
- **Leo Rising:** Highest energy in late summer, begins to retreat and turn inward in late winter
- **Virgo Rising:** Highest energy in early autumn, begins to retreat and turn inward in early spring
- **Libra Rising:** Highest energy at the autumn equinox, begins to retreat and turn inward at the spring equinox
- **Scorpio Rising:** Highest energy in late autumn, begins to retreat and turn inward in late spring
- **Sagittarius Rising:** Highest energy in early winter, begins to retreat and turn inward in early summer
- **Capricorn Rising:** Highest energy at the winter solstice, begins to retreat and turn inward at the summer solstice
- **Aquarius Rising:** Highest energy in late winter, begins to retreat and turn inward in late summer

- **Pisces Rising:** Highest energy in early spring, begins to retreat and turn inward in early autumn

At its most basic, you may be at your highest energy during the season of your ascendant sign and you're likely ready to retreat and turn inward during the season opposite of your ascendant. This is why some people are so in flow with the natural seasons, others are energized at the beginning of the new year, still others feel at their best when the crisp air of autumn rolls around, and so on. Your natural rhythms are also impacted by the rest of your chart and by your own experiences with the seasons, so this is not something to be taken at face value, but it's a great place to start getting more familiar with the way you interact with nature.

Not only can this information help you create seasonal self-care rituals that feel aligned and in flow but it can also help you prepare for the ebbs and flows of self-care in your life.

At the time of year when you are at your highest energy and for the three to four months following that season, your self-care practice is likely to be given renewed focus. This is when you're probably feeling at your best, and maybe least in *need* of self-care, but it's also when you have the most energy to give to the projects and ideas you're devoted to.

During your personal fall and winter, when you begin to wind down and eventually turn completely within, you're likely to be craving your self-care practice more to fill in the gaps in energy. Regardless of the actual seasons you experience these flows in, being aware of the way that your self-care practice needs to adapt to suit your needs is so important in sustaining your practice through the changes.

As your personal spring, the season of your ascendant sign, approaches, you will start to feel the energy building. Your excitement and enthusiasm for the coming season will be building up in you. This is a great time to make plans for your self-care practice, to consider what aspects you want to give fresh attention to and which things you want to let go of in this new season. Although you may very well feel like you don't need as much of a self-care practice during this time of high energy, it's the perfect time to experiment and play with what is really working for you. This is the time for adaptability and being open to change and fresh perspective in your rituals.

For me, as a Virgo Rising, my personal spring is Virgo season. I have the most energy and the most highly tuned focus (in all areas of life but especially in my spiritual and self-care practices), beginning in August and carrying me through about Halloween. It's the anticipation of the witches' season, the magick and moonlight of Halloween, but also of the fall weather, boots, and chai. (Yes, I'm kind of a basic witch when it comes to fall.)

As your personal summer approaches, the season approximately three months after the sun was in your ascendant sign, you will feel like basking in your self-care practice but you're also likely to feel more distracted from it as well. You probably feel a bit lazy-hazy, like you're happy and excited to be where you are but you also have so many fun things you *want* to do, that you often push your self-care or even spiritual practice to the back burner. And that's okay, it's just one of the seasonal rhythms. This is the time for fun and enjoyment—and for forgiving yourself when you fall off track.

For me, my personal summer is Sagittarius season, beginning in late November. I adore the holidays and for the period from

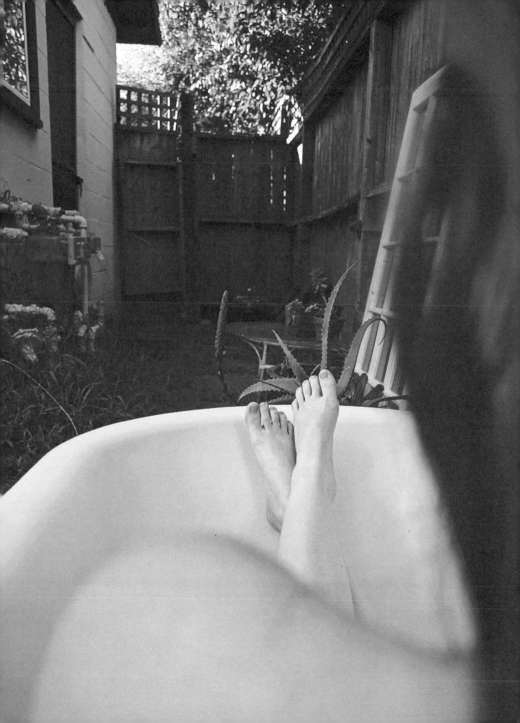

Thanksgiving through the Winter Solstice and even into the new year, I feel happy, bouncy, and joyful. But I also, without fail, load my schedule with things to do, people to see, parties to go to and to host. Unless I pay very close attention, I inevitably get off track with my self-care and often wind up getting sick in January because I haven't been taking caring of myself in the way I need to be.

As your personal autumn approaches, the season opposite from your ascendant sign, you are likely to begin wanting to retreat and withdraw. It's not the full retreat of winter, which is yet to come, but it's the deepening of shadows and the desire to spend more time alone. It's when you're curious about the inner work you could be doing. This is the time for gentleness and speaking especially kindly to yourself. It's a time for exploring shadows, to be sure.

For me, my personal autumn is Pisces season, beginning in late February, just before the actual spring equinox. It's a time when I'm self-reflective, when I want to define things and I start getting even a little anxious about my relationships and my choices. I start feeling like the new year is already slipping away from me and that I need to be taking action if I want to make my dreams happen. Translation: It's when my shadows start cropping up and I feel called to address them.

As your personal winter approaches, the season three signs or months prior to your ascendant sign, you begin the truly deep descent into retreat. If you suffer from depression or anxiety, this is the season when it is most likely to come up for you. This is less about shadow work and more about simply making your way out of the dark. This doesn't mean that your personal winter is a season to dread; in fact, there are many ways to make your personal winter a time of light and gentle celebration. During the actual winter, cultures all over the world have created celebrations of light. There is a quote from my favorite *Doctor Who* Christmas Special from 2010 (nerd flag flying) in which the narrator tells us, "On every world, wherever people are, in the deepest part of the winter, at the exact mid-point, everybody stops and turns and hugs. As if to say, 'Well done. Well done, everyone! We're halfway out of the dark.'" This is one of the most picturesque and oddly haunting descriptions of the winter solstice I've ever heard and one of the most accurate. Your personal winter is a time to find ways to celebrate being halfway out of the dark and to light up your life with joy and peace.

For me, my personal winter is Gemini season, carrying me through the rest of summer until we finally return to my rising sign of Virgo. The summer is definitely the most difficult time of year for me. I've always struggled with the blazing heat, the unstructured days, and the seemingly endless sunlight. That might make me sound like a downer, but it's not how I mean it at all: rather, as a Virgo rising, I just prefer the intimacy and coziness of autumn. It's not that I hate summer; in fact, there are many things I love about summer, from travel to beach days to stargazing.

Now is all of this to say that my natural rhythms and seasons are dictated by my astrological chart? No, of course not, and neither are yours. Although I adore fall and I definitely feel the renewed spirit in Virgo season, August, September, and October are also very difficult and emotional months for me. Late summer and early fall are what's known as fire season in California. Having lost my home in a wildfire in the month of September and been evacuated from multiple wildfires in the month of October, I experience very mixed feelings and a certain amount of depression at this time of year. Your natural rhythms are affected by your own life experiences, too, and getting intimate and honest with yourself about them will help you prepare the tools you need to thrive in all seasons.

You are also likely affected, to some degree, by the actual seasons as well, even if they are counterintuitive to your personal seasons. For example, a Capricorn Rising who loves the fresh start of the new year and the winter solstice, could still absolutely suffer from Seasonal Affective Disorder, experiencing depression and low energy due to the long nights and short, gray days of winter.

These seemingly counterintuitive combinations of seasonal experiences can make you feel a little like you're losing your mind at times. You might ask yourself at certain times of the year, how you can possibly feel both energized and excited, but still feel the fingers of depression as well?

The thing about self-care is that although practicing *any* amount of self-care is going to be supportive in some way, in order for it to be fully effective, your practice needs to be customized wholly to your own needs. We've been talking about this throughout this book but the often contradictory combination of the actual seasons and your personal seasons is the perfect opportunity to reinforce it. Take the time to pay attention, track your moods and emotions, track your energy levels, explore how you personally ebb and flow, and allow yourself to get curious about the contradictions.

Maybe your moods shift week to week, maybe there are some weeks in autumn when you feel full of renewed focus and other weeks when you feel low energy and motivation. Ask yourself why that could be. The answers to your own unique contradictions lie within you. Only you can answer those questions for yourself. Really think about what you've experienced in your life during each season of the year. How do those past experiences shape the way you feel now?

Think about how you were raised to view each season. Did your parents or siblings strongly favor one season over the others? Was that passed onto you, even though it may have been out of sync with your natural rhythms? Is that why you have mixed feelings about a particular season or another?

Think about your life in terms of events, as well. Are there particular things you do, places you go, or celebrations you attend during certain seasons? How do those events make you feel? Are they things you excitedly look forward to or are they dreaded? How does that shape the way you perceive and experience each season?

HOW TO PREPARE FOR SEASONS OF PLENTY

Spring and summer, both the actual seasons and your personal ones, depending on your relationship with them, are seasons of plenty. This is when we celebrate fertility, growth, rebirth, and the light of the sun. The days are long and the mood is jovial. This is theoretically when we experience our highest energy and our greatest desire to *do things*.

Preparing for spring and summer in terms of your self-care practice is a matter of making space for fun. Adapting your rituals so that they are shorter, less structured, and give you time for spontaneity is important. Mini-rituals are a great way to keep your self-care practice in place, while allowing yourself the space to not have to feel guilty when you're distracted by fun adventures and inspiring projects.

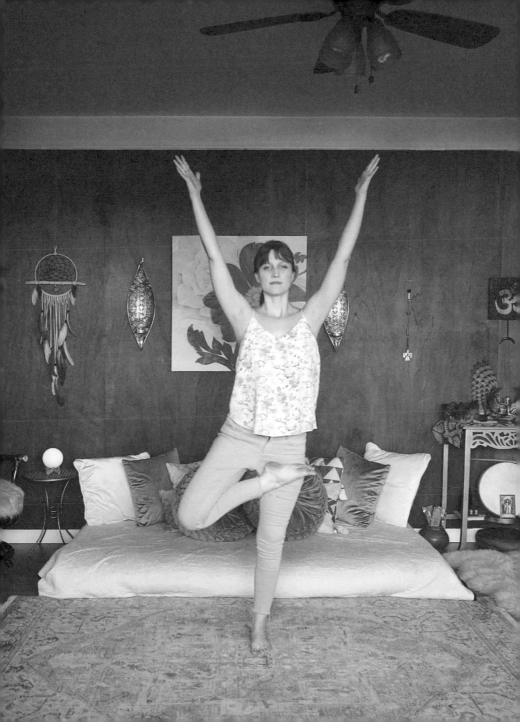

Once you've identified your core feelings around each season, even if they are contradictory, you will be able to prepare for the ebbs and flows of emotion and energy that come with each.

The purpose of your self-care practice at any time of year, at its heart, is to provide a space in which you never have to feel guilty. You never have to feel like you didn't accomplish what you set out to, because the only thing your self-care practice needs to accomplish is being supportive.

HOW TO PREPARE FOR SEASONS OF SHADOW

Autumn and winter, again, both the actual seasons and your personal ones, are seasons of shadow. This is when we celebrate our roots and give thanks for everything that gives us life and sustains us when we delve deep into our shadows and explore who we are at our core. The nights are long and the mood is intimate. This is theoretically when we experience our lowest energy but our deepest transformations.

Preparing for autumn and winter in your self-care is about creating a support system for yourself. This is the time when you probably have more time to spend at home and when you desire to hibernate. When you want to curl up with that cup of tea and a good book and just be alone with your thoughts. It's of the utmost importance to adapt your rituals so that they're deeply nourishing and give you the support you need when you *don't* feel highly motivated, so that you don't have to feel guilty about that either.

Sustainability may not sound like a very sexy concept, but creating rituals that can weather any storm of your life will turn your spiritual and self-care practices into a stronger foundation to express yourself from. Whatever it is that could potentially keep you from practicing self-care or expressing your spirituality, ignoring it is only giving it power over you.

In fact, it's time for some real talk. It doesn't matter what is making your life feel so crazy: whether you need a better work/life balance, you suffer from chronic illness, or you simply get overwhelmed by the daily tasks of work and family (and the endless washing of dishes and laundry that is adulting). Whatever it is, pretending that all of those things are suddenly going to cease being a problem for you just because you've created some self-care rituals is not going to get you anywhere. Your self-care rituals are not a magickal Band-Aid that's going to somehow give you more hours in the day.

Well, then, so what's the point?

Self-care is not a fix-it solution; it's a foundation to help you create a more magickal life. Giving yourself space to create variations on your rituals and to create a practice that exists in *flow* and alignment with your natural rhythms, these are the tools you need to create the life you want. One where dishes and laundry still exist, but you don't feel so overwhelmed by needing to do them. A life where you still have challenges but you're better equipped to face them, and where you know how to speak kindly to yourself when those challenges arise.

Chapter 7

SELF-CARE RITUALS FOR YOUR MIND & BODY

Caring for your mind and body is the first step in practicing spiritual self-care. If your physical, mental, and emotional needs are not met, it will be a struggle to progress to the next stages of enlightenment.

We see throughout history, *almost* universally, that humans first learned to tame the land and animals, then began to create portable art like pottery. It is only after we stopped being hunter-gatherers that we had the time and capacity to create beautiful objects. It is also after settlement began that we became philosophers and to ponder the big questions of the universe.

Once our most basic needs are met, we discover that there is more space within us than we could have ever imagined.

It is the same with self-care. When we are constantly in survival mode, constantly straining to eat healthy, to exercise, to feel connected to and grounded in our bodies, to feel nourished and supported, to feel safe expressing our emotions . . . we struggle to create beauty in other areas of our lives.

That's why a well-rounded and transformative spiritual self-care practice must begin with the mind and body. It is important to remember, though, that the mind and body are your most accessible tools for creating magick, only when they are cared for. The rituals on the following pages will support you in caring for these basic needs in a way that also acknowledges that your mind and body are more than simply vessels for your spirit.

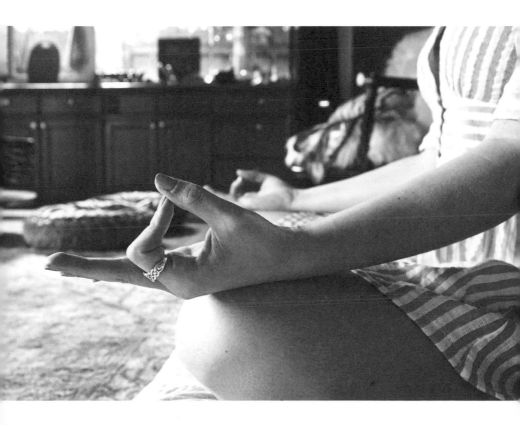

A Witchy Meditation to Ease Anxiety

Meditation is perhaps one of the most obvious ways to care for your mind, since it is an act that takes place entirely *within* your mind! You don't need any tools to practice magick, witchcraft, or self-care of any kind but meditation really takes the cake with this one—truly all you need to meditate is yourself. Practicing meditation and mindfulness, being in the moment, has been shown to reduce anxiety and ease stress. Hence the rise of popular meditation apps and even guided meditations to download from your favorite influencers!

A lot of people are still automatically turned off by the idea of meditation, though, because they've tried sitting still, quieting their minds, and being silent, and just find themselves thinking about their grocery list for ten minutes instead. If this is you, never fear—of course there are witchy ways to meditate that may align more with your needs while still easing anxiety!

When we experience "negative" emotions like anxiety, what we're really feeling is an elemental imbalance. For a witch, the elements rule all aspects of life, and bringing them back into balance through meditation and magick is an excellent way to gain relief.

The mind and mental health are ruled by the element of air, so to ease anxiety and other stresses, we'll bring in water and earth in this meditation for balance.

You Will Need:

Just yourself, of course! But, if you'd like to use some meditation aids, here are a few suggestions:

- Relaxing incense such as cedarwood or essential oils such as lavender

- A soft pillow or cushion to sit on
- Soft instrumental music

Set up your space at your altar however you prefer. Light the incense or apply diluted essential oils to your temple and wrists. Just get comfy.

Close your eyes and place your hands on your knees or belly. Acknowledge the anxiety and stress that is currently plaguing you. Take a step outside of yourself to acknowledge the anxiety coiled within you. It's okay that it's there.

Feel the weight of your body on the ground or chair beneath you. Starting at the top of your head, slowly do a mental scan of your entire body. When you reach the bottoms of your feet, imagine roots leaving your body and driving down into the earth below. The earth is here to support you.

A full moon moves into view above your head. It shines down on you, becoming a pulsing stream of light that moves into your body and permeates your entire being. The light becomes concentrated around your heart, spinning and swirling around it so your chest feels warm and content. The moon is here to support you.

Stay here, rooted to the earth and nurtured by the moon, as long as you need. When you are ready, imagine the roots slowly withdrawing back into your body and the light subsiding into your heart. You will carry these protective energies with you as you move into the rest of your day.

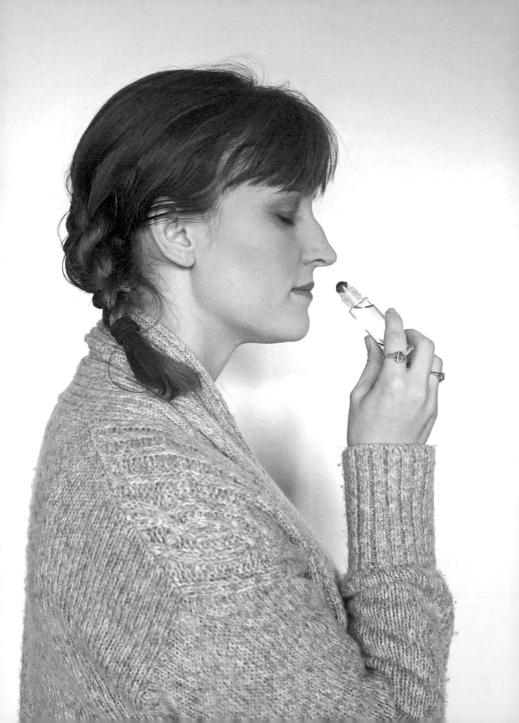

Aromatherapy Oil Blend for Clearing the Mind

Sometimes we all need a little support in clearing our heads. We get cluttered with thoughts, to-do lists, worries, fears, and stray distractions. When it's time to focus on your self-care practice or to work a little magick, it can be difficult to clear your head and give your full attention to what's at hand.

This aromatherapy blend of essential oils is designed for exactly those moments. You can either combine the oils in your diffuser whenever you please or create a roller ball blend to inhale as needed.

RECIPE FOR DIFFUSER BLEND

- 4 drops lemon oil for purification
- 3 drops angelica oil for healing visions
- 2 drops juniper oil for love and protection
- 2 drops spearmint oil for banishing mental chatter

Whenever you feel mentally cluttered and need a moment of peace and serenity, place this blend in your diffuser. Take the time to make this act a ritual. Carefully and mindfully fill the diffuser with water as directed and think about the magickal intent of each oil as you place its drops in the diffuser.

Breathe deeply as you turn on the diffuser and allow the molecules to calm and center you.

RECIPE FOR ROLLER BALL BLEND

- 6 drops lemon oil for purification
- 4 drops angelica oil for healing visions
- 3 drops juniper oil for love and protection
- 3 drops spearmint oil for banishing mental chatter

Fill the rest of the bottle with carrier oil of your choice such as coconut oil and cap with roller ball.

If you opt for a roller ball of this blend, you can take it with you wherever you go! Whether you need mental clarity before a larger ritual or just in the middle of the day, uncap your roller ball with intention and close your eyes. Breathe deeply from the bottle and allow it to work its magick!

However you prefer to work with essential oils, this blend is intended to aid you in not only clearing your mind and banishing chatter and negative thoughts but also to invite in love and healing visions of what is possible.

Social Media Detox

Most of us have been guilty of the social media scroll hole at some point. You've sat there in bed or on the couch, scrolling through your Instagram, Facebook, or Pinterest feed and when you look up, you're shocked to discover that an hour has passed. Once in a while, an hour of mindlessness can be supportive in helping us disconnect from the stresses of the day.

Neanderthals probably cursed the invention of the wheel too, but we all came to cope with that one. I actually believe modern technology is a blessing, allowing us to connect to people all around the globe who have all sorts of incredible ideas and inspirations. But all that screen time, waking up and immediately looking at our phones, and the disconnection from human interaction has taken a toll on our society. They say we don't know how to make legitimate human connection anymore and that we don't know how to be bored, always reaching for our phones in even a few seconds of downtime. That's why a social media detox can be super powerful in helping you to make space in your mind for *you* to exist. Unplugging can help you to realize that your mind is packed with ideas and insights that you just can't hear when technology is in the way.

Think of a social media detox as a sort of cleansing ritual for the mind. Just as you might burn sage to purify your home, turn your phone off to purify your mind! I can't say I'm great at this but when you give yourself something to replace the technology attachment with, it works far better than trying to go cold turkey for a day or even an hour. Replacing your digital inundation with a ritual is the perfect alternative.

Begin by deciding how long you'd like to unplug for. It could be an hour, six hours, a day, however long feels right. Plan in advance what you will do with your time while you're unplugged. Maybe there's a book you've had on your nightstand for months, just waiting to be read, or maybe you've been craving some time out in nature for a walk or a yoga practice.

Turn off all your readily available devices, like your smartphone,

HOW TO USE PINTEREST FOR GOOD!

Pinterest may be the ultimate time suck but did you know it's actually perfect for creating vision boards and virtual altars?

Pinterest gets lumped in with the social media platforms like Facebook and Instagram but it's actually a search engine. Far more efficient and eco-friendly than cutting pictures out of magazines, Pinterest grants access to all the beautiful images of the Internet.

Create "secret" boards that only you can see and pin images of your ideal life to create a vision board. This could focus on career, body image, your physical reality (such as your home), or even how you express yourself as a witch.

You can also create a virtual altar to honor a particular concept or even a planet or deity by pinning images to a board that represent the symbols, colors, and energy of what you wish to express devotion for.

Although we talk a lot about needing to detox from social media and about the toxicity of being so immersed in social expectations all the time, there are positives to every social media platform. Unless you're planning to go completely off the grid, it's unlikely that you can avoid social media or technology entirely and I don't believe you should. Rather, find ways to express your spirituality and to practice self-care through social media instead!

tablet, and laptop, and place them in one spot, preferably in a room you won't be going into much for the duration of your detox. (If you need to have a phone on for others to contact you, it's fine to keep it with you—there are apps you can download to specifically repress access to social media!)

Now, go to your altar and find a comfortable place to sit or lie down. Light some candles and incense or put on your essential oil diffuser. Close your eyes, and just listen to yourself. Allow your own voice to come through. Often, we don't allow this to happen because we don't want to hear the thoughts we know will come. The voice of self-doubt, ridicule, and sabotage. The voice that says we aren't good enough or we aren't loved enough. It's okay if those thoughts come. Just be aware of their existence and allow them to fade away. So many of those fears of not being enough in some way (good enough, smart enough, pretty enough, fit enough), come from our intense immersion in toxic social media. The point here is not to listen for the voice of your ego but rather to listen for the voice of your intuition. Your intuition is always there, it's always right, and it always has supportive insight for you, if you're willing to listen.

I recommend practicing this active, intuitive listening for ten to fifteen minutes to start and then going about the rest of your detox with the activities you planned previously, such as reading, going for a walk, cooking a meal, journaling, or just spending time with loved ones.

Make time for an intentional and intuitive social media detox periodically so that you can take this opportunity to strengthen your intuition and become more aware of what your true inner voice sounds like. When you are familiar with that inner voice, it becomes easier to clear your mind and listen for it when you really need to.

Bubble Bath to Soothe the Soul

We've been talking about why bubble baths are not the ultimate form of self-care all throughout this book; it's time we talked about why bubble baths can be pretty great, too!

When self-care became commercialized and trendy, bubble baths shot to the forefront of the industry. Companies began making all sorts of luxurious bath products to take your bath to the next level. And there's actually nothing whatsoever wrong with that: having bath bombs and herbal soaks that smell great and introduce an element of magick can be an awesome way to relax and unwind. As always, though, you don't need any tools to perform a ritual bath, only your body and a tub of water (warm or cool, depending on your purposes).

Like many forms of commercialized self-care, bubble baths have also taken on a connotation of laziness. If you have time to lounge about all day in the bath, eating chocolates, and reading a book, then you somehow aren't fulfilling your social obligations. This negative portrayal is meant to guilt-trip you into believing that your self-care practice is a selfish act. On the other hand, since most of us don't have time to lounge about all day in the bath, we can feel guilty about not living up to this portrayal either!

With these classic images of self-care, we have to untangle the true depth of meaning from all these layers of social guilt. Bathing is actually one of the most ancient forms of ritual. It was a sacred practice in Ancient Greece and Rome and was even a way to honor some goddesses, like Venus.

Let's take a look at why: first of all, nudity is sacred. Clothes are contraptions contrived by man to meet our expectations of beauty and modesty (and to practically protect us from the elements), but our nude bodies are expressions of the divine, and spending time getting to know your body is a sacred act. Plus, the physical act of bathing is a grounding practice. Touching your skin, cleaning it, and giving it attention helps you get in touch with the physical world—and the physical world is only a reflection of the spiritual one and vice versa.

That's why this bubble bath is about grounding, soothing your soul, and getting in touch with the divine—but feel free to eat some chocolate and read a book while you're in there, too!

You Will Need:

- Your favorite bubble bath
- A bundle of fresh lavender for soothing
- Emerald or green calcite crystals for grounding
- Candles

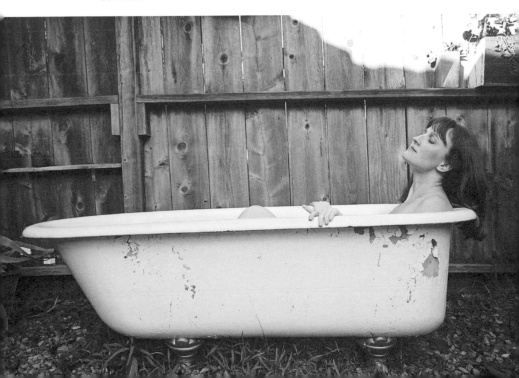

Hang the bundle of fresh lavender over the faucet of the tub so it hangs behind where the water comes out. As the steam rises from the hot water, it will release the soothing scent of the lavender.

Let the water run until it reaches your desired temperature, then plug the drain and pour a capful of your favorite bubble bath into the running water.

Allow the tub to fill, then shut off the water. Place the crystals around the outside of the tub. Light a few candles and place these around the tub as well. Turn out the lights and be sure to have a towel and bath mat readily available for when you are finished.

Relax into the bath and allow your eyes to close. Regardless of what obligations you have to fulfill when you leave this space, this moment is just for you.

Press your hands together in a prayer position and really feel the weight of your fingers and palms pushing against each other. Move the fingers of your right hand down over your left wrist and mindfully touch your arm. Allow your hands to move over your arms, shoulders, chest, torso, hips, thighs, calves, feet.

Touch your body mindfully and with intention, grounding into the sensation of being a person with a physical body on this physical earth.

Release your breath out with a sigh and sink back in the tub. Allow your body to fully and consciously relax. Stay in the bath as long as you can. Extinguish the candles when you get out.

Moon Salutations Yin Yoga Flow

I like to begin my own rituals with movement. I find it to be grounding and it helps me to get in the right mindset for magick and ritual as well. It's hard to think about anything else when you're holding a yoga pose and focusing on your breath, especially when practicing yin yoga.

Yin is a form of yoga in which the yogi or yogini holds each pose for an extended amount of time and poses are focused on gentle, stretching motions. Yin yoga practitioners might hold a single yoga pose for up to five to ten minutes, as opposed to the thirty second rule of thumb in the fast-paced vinyasa yoga you may be used to!

The idea of yin yoga is to really focus on deep relaxation and allowing the body to sink into each pose. In many cases, the longer you hold a pose, the more opportunity you have to relax into it and to receive its benefits. It's a very emotional and spiritual form of yoga that can serve as a relaxing type of meditation as well.

The following suggested yin yoga flow is inspired by the phases of the moon and is an answer to the classic sun salutations. Sun salutations are a sequence of yoga poses designed to wake the body up, warm up the muscles, and connect to the breath before beginning a full practice or as a quick practice on their own. Moon salutations do the opposite: these sequences of poses are used to calm the mind and relax the body. These are great sequences to do right before bed or before a longer ritual as they are really grounding and centering but also open the heart.

You can practice moon salutations at whatever speed you are most comfortable with. Thirty seconds per pose is perfectly acceptable but when you find yourself in a space where you know you need

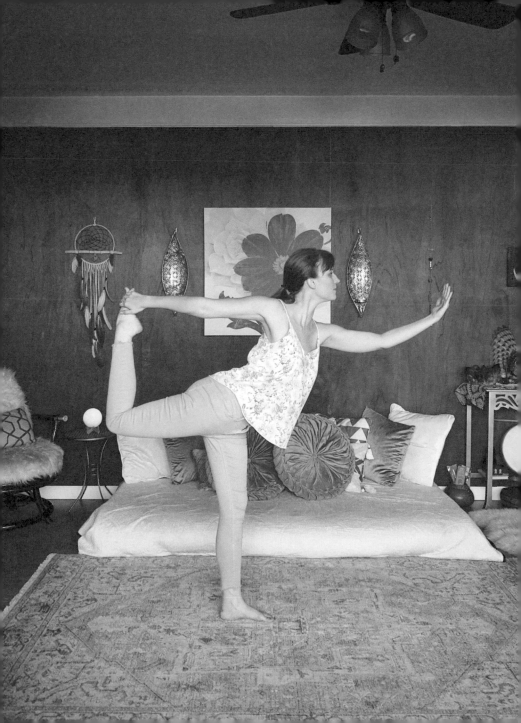

to listen to your body more, I recommend trying out the yin yoga practice of holding each pose for at least two to three minutes. This gives you a chance to really feel what's happening in your body and to consciously relax each muscle. Think of it like an active savasana!

To begin, roll out your mat and set up your space so it feels inviting and cozy. Consider lighting some candles, laying out a soft blanket and pillows beside your mat, and turning on some gentle instrumental music that puts your mind at ease. At any point during your yin practice, you can lay the blanket over your body, rest your head on the pillow, or tuck it under your hips or knees. I also like to put a pot of tea on to brew while I practice so it's warm and ready to sip when I'm finished.

Stand at the head of your mat in mountain pose and take a full, deep breath in through the nose, lifting your arms overhead. Release the breath out through your mouth and bring your hands to your heart in prayer pose. Consciously drop your shoulders. Allow your eyes to close. Breathe in and out a few times.

When you are ready, raise your arms over head again and fold over. Come to your knees and sink back into child's pose. If you would like, you can rest your head on a pillow here. Hold this pose for thirty seconds up to five minutes. This pose represents the dark or new phase of the moon, when it is completely dark in the night sky.

Lift your body slightly and touch your toes together, moving your knees apart to the edges of your mat and reaching your arms overhead for wide child's pose. Hold this pose for thirty seconds up to five minutes.

Pull yourself up and forward, reaching your toes back to plank position. Hold this pose for ten seconds up to three minutes.

Slowly and carefully lower yourself down, keeping your elbows in, and rest your entire body for reverse savasana pose. Lay your cheek or forehead on the mat and rest your arms down alongside your body. Hold this pose for thirty seconds up to five minutes.

Place your hands on the mat beneath your shoulders and press your upper body up into cobra pose. Hold this pose for thirty seconds to five minutes. These poses represent the waxing crescent moon as it begins to appear in the sky.

Press your thighs back and push yourself up into downward dog pose. Lift your hips to the sky and lower your heels toward the mat. Step your right foot forward between your hands into a low lunge. Lift your arms overhead and lean back into a gentle low lunge with backbend, reaching toward the wall behind you. Hold this pose for thirty seconds up to five minutes. This pose represents the waxing moon as it approaches the first quarter.

Lower your hands to the mat on either side of your foot and step your left leg in to meet your right so you are in a standing forward bend. Sweeping your arms up, rise to stand in mountain pose.

Place your hands on your lower back and lower your shoulder blades down your back, bending into a standing supported backbend. Hold this pose for ten seconds up to two minutes.

Lift your upper body back to straight, finding mountain pose again. Load your right foot and lift your left foot into the crease of your right hip for half lotus tree. Lift your arms overhead. Hold this pose for ten seconds up to five minutes. These poses represent the waxing quarter moon, when half the face of the moon is visible in the sky.

Lower your left foot back to the floor and find mountain pose again. Load your right foot again and kick your left foot into your left hand. Raise your right arm overhead and lean forward, lifting your left leg in the air behind you for king dancer pose. Hold this pose for ten seconds up to five minutes.

Lean back to standing straight and lower your left foot back to the floor, finding mountain pose again. Turn to face the side of your mat and place your hands on your hips. Separate your feet apart and turn your toes slightly inward. Bend over slowly and place your hands on the mat for wide-legged forward fold. Hold this pose for thirty seconds to five minutes. These poses represent the waxing gibbous moon, as the moon waxes toward full.

Return your hands to your hips and lift yourself back up to standing. Bend your knees out and lift your arms up at a ninety-degree angle on either side of your body so your upper arms are parallel with your thighs. Lower your shoulder blades and square your arms and legs for goddess pose. Hold this pose for thirty seconds to five minutes. This pose represents the full moon in all her magick and light.

For the second half of the sequence, move through all of the poses in reverse order to represent the waning moon: wide-legged forward fold, mountain, king dancer (left leg standing), mountain, half lotus tree (left leg standing), mountain, standing supported backbend, mountain, standing forward bend, low lunge with backbend (left leg forward), cobra, reverse savasana, plank, child's pose.

Body Crystal Grid for Grounding

My personal favorite way to work with crystals is literally just holding them. Feeling the cool crystal on my hands or skin, meditating with them, or using them to choose tarot cards, I find the feel and weight of them very soothing. Crystals are naturally grounding because they come from the earth and they make excellent allies for connecting more with your body.

A crystal grid is really just that: an assortment of crystals laid out in a carefully crafted grid. Crystal grids are used to charge items with magickal intent or to boost the power of a particular intention that you've set. Crystal grids can be very complex and form beautiful mandalas or just a few special stones laid out in a comforting way.

I love to work with crystal grids on the body because it connects you so viscerally to the earth and supercharges you with grounded energy!

You Will Need:

- 3–8 crystals of your choosing

Lay down in a comfortable place. You may want to put on some soft music, burn incense and candles, or diffuse some essential oils.

Place the first crystal on your forehead to activate your third eye.

Optionally, you may also place crystals over your throat, heart, solar plexus, sacral, and root chakras (on the throat, heart, low rib cage, naval, and low belly).

Hold at least one crystal in each hand and rest your arms on either side of your body. Close your eyes.

Envision light surrounding each of the crystals on your body, beginning with the one on your forehead. Consciously feel the weight of the crystal on your body. Picture that light circling you in a warm, comforting way and then send that light down into the earth below you, connecting you to your roots. Repeat this visualization with each crystal you've used.

When you have completed the visualization with each crystal, return to your body, feeling your weight on the surface beneath you and the light pressure of each crystal on your skin. When you are ready, open your eyes.

SUGGESTED CRYSTALS FOR GROUNDING WORK

- Obsidian
- Green calcite
- Desert rose
- Smoky quartz
- Moss agate

Chapter 8
SELF-CARE RITUALS FOR NOURISHING YOUR INTUITION

Your intuition is a tool that you carry with you, just as your mind and body are. It is inseparable from who you are as a person and as a witch. Getting in touch with, learning to understand, and really trusting your intuition are somewhat more challenging than trusting your own thoughts or the physical sensations you feel in your body, though.

We have been conditioned *not* to trust our intuition. Especially as women, we are often dismissed by medical professionals about what we intuitively know to be true about our bodies. We're expected to do something practical and socially acceptable with our lives—everyone pursuing an art degree knows what it's like to be quizzed about how you're going to make money. God forbid you follow your heart. People of every gender are ridiculed for studying tarot or astrology. They get asked, "you don't *really* believe in that sort of thing, do you?"

This isn't really a new phenomenon. The Age of Enlightenment, a period in the 1700s that brought science and reason to the forefront of western culture, did us many favors. It led to scientific breakthroughs and a greater understanding of the human mind. It led to the foundation of democracies and even to the end of the witch trials throughout Europe and the Americas because most people no longer believed in witchcraft.

What the Age of Enlightenment cost us is the belief in ourselves. Witchcraft may have no longer been a hanging offense in most European countries by the dawn of the nineteenth century but it became a subject of ridicule instead or, at best, a parlor trick.

Yet divination tools have been used literally since the dawn of time. Only in the last few hundred years have these intuitive tools become little more than a game, with the *tarocchi* of fifteenth-century Italy and similar games appearing in France and Austria. As modern witches, it's our job to recapture the intuitive wisdom of our ancestors and start nourishing our intuition again.

It's no accident that the Pluto in Scorpio generation (otherwise known as millennials) are bringing tools like tarot, pendulums, and dream journaling back into mainstream culture. Pluto is the planet of the witch and it was in its home sign of Scorpio from 1983 to 1995. Scorpio rules the occult, witchcraft, and all things taboo, including divination. Our renewed interest as a generation in the occult and divination is cosmically designed. It's literally our purpose to come together to bring these traditions back into the mainstream.

So what does this newly resurrected fascination with divination have to do with self-care?

As you learned early on in this book, relying on your intuition is essential for developing a self-care practice that actually fulfills your own unique needs. Being able to listen to and trust your intuition depends on knowing what your intuition sounds like, knowing how to recognize when you're receiving an intuitive hit, and knowing that you can trust yourself 100 percent, even when the answers you receive from your higher self seem out of sync with your ego or social expectations.

On the following pages, you'll find ideas and inspiration to nourish your intuition every day!

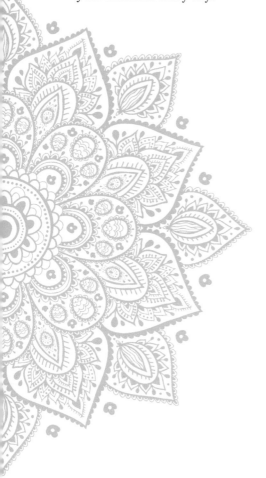

Enlightening Tea Blend to Awaken Your Intuition

Whatever your preferred divination tools are, however you like to connect with and listen to your intuition, and no matter how advanced you are with intuitive work, sometimes it's just difficult to tune out the world and tune into your higher self.

Having a ritual that helps you flip the switch from your mundane day-to-day experiences to a fully connected expression of your inner witch can be really helpful.

I love to work with specific tea blends that I only drink during certain moon phases, on certain seasonal celebrations, or for certain magickal workings. It really helps put me in the right mindset for expressing my spirituality in that moment.

This blend is designed to help you flip that switch and awaken your intuition with the very first sip so that you can be fully aligned and ready to listen to the messages your higher self has for you! Drink it before your next tarot reading, scrying session, or even right before bed to encourage prophetic dreams.

Ingredients:

- 1 tablespoon white tea leaves
- 1 teaspoon dried lavender flowers
- 1 teaspoon dried jasmine flowers
- 1 teaspoon dried mugwort

Combine all ingredients in a tea infuser or tea bag and place in mug. Pour hot water over and allow to steep for two to three minutes.

Get comfy at your altar or somewhere peaceful where you can access your divination tools. (I like to sit in bed and read my cards!)

Allow yourself space to sip your tea and relax into the moment before moving into your divination ritual.

Taking this extra five minutes for yourself can really put you in the right mindset to receive even more powerful intuitive downloads!

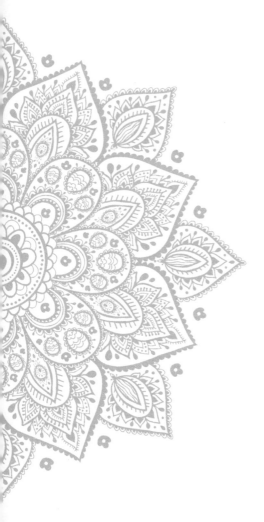

Working with Tarot and Oracle Cards

Tarot is a system of divination by card reading. There are many possibilities for its origin, but it probably became popular within the occult in the eighteenth century. Within a tarot deck, there are twenty-two major arcana cards and fifty-six minor arcana cards.

The major arcana are those you may be most familiar with, including the fool, death, hanged man, lovers, and hermit cards. In a reading, these typically indicate major life events or big life lessons to learn.

The minor arcana might sound more like a deck of playing cards at first glance: there are four suits (wands, pentacles, swords, and cups), and each suit features a king, queen, knight, page, ace, and numbers two through ten. Each suit is ruled by one of the elements, and in a reading these cards typically represent how something will happen, the people you will interact with, or the way that you need to show up in order to bring what you desire into reality.

Tarot cards can be read completely intuitively but each card does have a traditional meaning, as well as an additional or opposite meaning when the card appears upside down (called "reversed"). Most tarot readers that I know and work with have studied the traditional meanings and incorporate them into their intuitive readings.

Oracle cards are a more modern phenomenon. There are no hard-and-fast rules about what comprises an oracle deck. They can be any shape and feature any number of cards with any thematic titles. I have oracle decks with traditional suits like the tarot, a circular deck that draws on the moon signs and phases for inspiration, and decks that are mostly prized for their beautiful artwork. Oracle decks often have a theme and might have affirmations or mantras on each card or just a phrase or word.

Because every oracle deck is different, there are no traditional meanings for each card. Some decks may come with a book that explains what each card means but oracle card readings are usually very intuitive, the word or phrase on each card sparking inspiration and understanding about the topic.

Neither tarot nor oracle cards are "better" than the other. The only thing that matters is that you feel connected to the deck you're working with and that you can trust your intuition to guide you in a reading. Personally, I mostly prefer to work with oracle cards in my own practice and have a few favorite decks in particular, but incorporate tarot into my readings and rituals as I feel called to do so.

On the following pages, you will find rituals for working with your cards as well as two card spreads to guide you in getting in touch with and trusting your intuition.

One common myth is that you cannot buy an oracle or tarot deck for yourself, but rather that they must always be gifted to you. Essentially, the idea is that the right deck will come to you when it is time and so going out and buying one you like is not as powerful as being given one. This is an old belief and one that some people still hold, but it's only true if it is true for you.

Your first challenge for nourishing your intuition is to ask yourself if this is a belief that is true for you, that a tarot deck must be given and not purchased . . . and to trust that the answer you receive from within, whatever it is, is 100 percent correct!

A daily card reading is a great way to nurture your intuition every day but sometimes a more in-depth reading can go a long way in breaking through blocks. In these cases, a tarot or oracle card spread is an ideal way to read multiple cards at once for maximum impact!

The following two spreads will support you in trusting your intuitive wisdom. You can draw either tarot or oracle cards for these spreads, or a combination of both! Whatever you feel called to do.

SPREAD FOR GETTING IN TOUCH WITH YOUR INTUITION

This spread is ideal for the newbie witch who is struggling to recognize when she is receiving an intuitive hit, but it will also be supportive for those who just need a boost in reconnecting with their intuition as well.

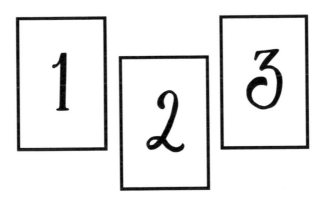

Card 1: Where is the source of my intuitive wisdom rooted?

Card 2: What does the voice of my intuition sound like?

Card 3: How can I practically channel my intuition in any situation?

SPREAD FOR LEARNING TO TRUST YOUR INTUITION

It is one thing to know what your intuition sounds like or where you feel intuitive nudges in your body. It's another thing entirely to actually know that the wisdom you are receiving is correct, trustworthy, and in your best interest. This spread is designed to help you learn to trust your intuition on a deep, soul level so that you can take action in your life without fear (whether it's taking action to create a self-care practice, to make a change in your career or relationship, or anything else that feels scary and uncertain).

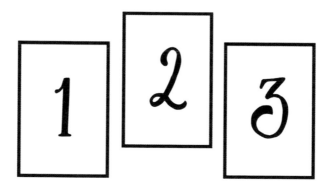

Card 1: How can I be certain that information I receive from my intuition is always in my best interest?

Card 2: How can I show up in a way that allows my intuition to speak first, before my ego or conditioning, so that I know my first instincts are always right?

Card 3: What is one message I need to hear from my higher self right now to demonstrate the power of my intuition?

In addition to this spread, I encourage you to reflect back on times when your intuition *was* right. This is a great journaling exercise, to record instances when you trusted your intuition, took action based on it, and saw success or growth in life because of it. This internal proof is sometimes the most powerful way to begin trusting your intuition—and yourself.

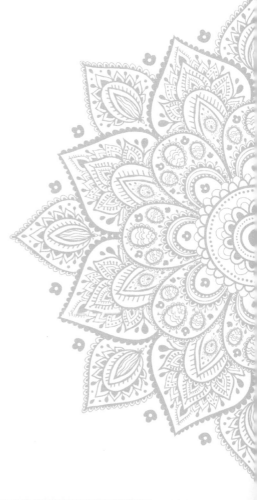

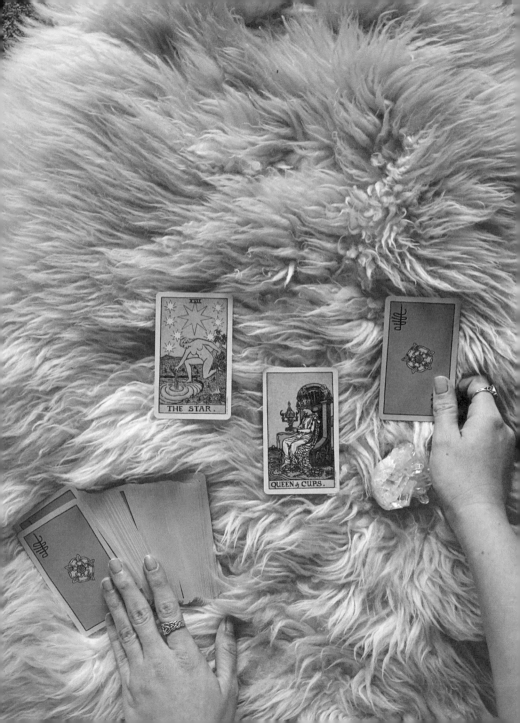

Tarot Journaling

Another excellent way to work with the cards is to keep a tarot or oracle card journal. Journaling and self-reflection are perhaps the ultimate self-care tools because they allow you to record your thoughts and feelings in any given moment and then look back on them in the future. This is true of simple daily journaling of your thoughts but it's also true when you use journaling in specific scenarios, such as nature journaling, dream journaling—or tarot journaling!

A tarot journal can be set up in a number of different ways to support your divination journey and is easily adapted for however you want to use it. The purpose of this journal is to help you get more comfortable with the cards themselves and with using them to tap into your intuition. You can use a plain lined notebook for this or a binder so that you can add and reorganize as needed.

Here are a few ideas for organizing and utilizing your tarot journal:

Create a section for getting intimate with each tarot card or with each card in a particular oracle deck:
Write out a list of the cards in order at the beginning of the section and number the following pages sequentially. When working with your journal, choose a particular card from the list or work through them in order. Sift through your deck to find that card and study it carefully.

You can record anything about the card in your tarot journal: what the symbols and imagery bring to mind for you and any inspiration about what the card would mean for you in a reading. In some ways you are creating a new reference book for the deck, based on your own intuition, as well as getting more intimately familiar with the meaning of each card.

Record your daily card reading:
Drawing a card every day is a great way to hone your intuition and receive wisdom from your higher self on a daily basis. I find that when I not only draw a card every day but record which card I drew and do a little journaling about it, patterns begin to emerge that I might not have noticed otherwise.

I often get asked what it means when you draw the same card over and over again on a regular basis. This happens to me too and it can be both frustrating and enlightening. When I was waiting for things to fall into place so that I could leave my full-time job and step fully into my career as a professional witch, I drew the "patience" card from one of my favorite oracle decks every few days. I was antsy and anxious for the situation to move forward but that card kept just consistently reminding me of what was really needed.

Now, looking back, I have rarely drawn that card since moving on from that particular situation.

Track common themes, recurring suits, or ruling elements of the cards you draw each day:
One thing that can be interesting to track is the element of the cards you draw every day. With tarot decks in particular, each suit is ruled by a different element, and some oracle decks are organized in this way as well. Whenever I track the elemental ruler of my daily card, I find that certain elements are strongest for me during particular times of my life.

A lot of fire cards might indicate a need to take action or express your passions more.

A lot of earth cards might indicate a need for grounding and looking at a situation more practically.

A lot of air cards might indicate a need for creative expression or getting out of the box.

A lot of water cards might indicate a need for listening to your intuition or expressing your emotions more.

Of course, if a particular element is conspicuously absent, there can be important lessons to be found there as well!

Recording your daily card draw is great for self-reflection, too, because you can always look back on which cards and elements you were drawing regularly at certain times in your life. It can be so supportive to see what you were once struggling with and how you evolved out of that situation into the person you are now. Alternatively, it can also be supportive to realize that you are still struggling with some of the same things and that perhaps now is the time to give those struggles your full attention.

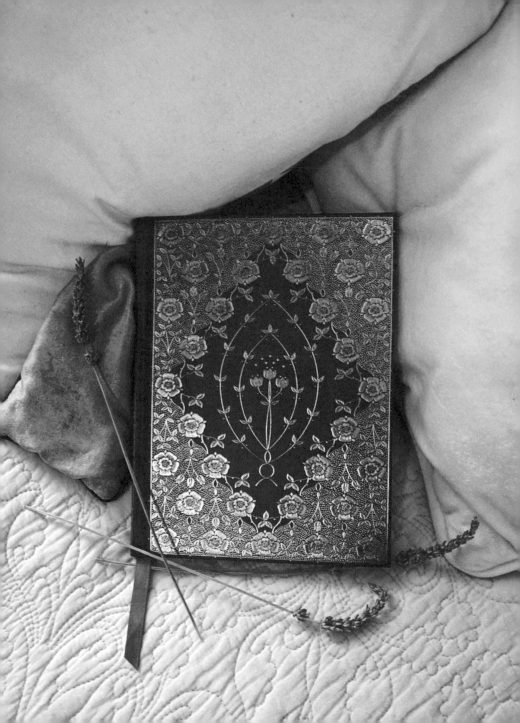

Getting Deeper with Dream Journaling

Back in Chapter 2 on page 34, we learned about dream journaling and how to start a daily practice with it. As with many things, though, getting started is one thing and maintaining a practice is often something else altogether.

Dream journaling is a great introduction to intuitive work because it's so accessible. After a few weeks or months of writing down your dreams every day, you will probably feel more connected and self-aware than ever before. But even after a significant period of this, some people still struggle to remember their dreams. Others are simply sure that most of the dreams they have are fairly meaningless or just don't make any sense.

The fact of the matter is that not all intuitive practices are for everyone. If dream journaling is not your cup of tea, you may need to find other rituals to nourish your intuition. If you do (intuitively) know that dream journaling is for you, though, but have just become bored with it or continue to struggle with connecting to it, then the following ritual and ideas will assist you in getting deeper with dream journaling.

As you may have gathered in reading this book, I'm a very practical witch. (Taurus sun, here.) Although when you first get started with dream journaling, it feels like stepping into a magickal portal to a world where you have psychic powers (and in many ways, it is . . .) the real power of dream journaling is in the act of self-reflection.

You can write down your dreams every morning, reflect on what they might mean, and then go about your day, never really thinking about them again and that can still be a valuable way to bring awareness to your intuition. But if you go back periodically, once a week or once a month or even once a year, and read back through your dream journal, you will discover deeper patterns of messages than you could ever really notice in the moment.

I am always amazed how when I read old dreams, even dreams I recorded years earlier, I'm often transported right into the visuals of that dream again. This doesn't happen every time, sometimes I don't remember the dream at all, but I often remember them in exquisite detail, especially those transformative, deeply coded dreams that were coming straight from my intuition.

I also discover patterns in those old journals. Themes that recur in my life that I've been struggling with in the present—but that I already struggled with and worked through once or several times in the past. It's brought me self-awareness about so many deeply ingrained beliefs that I intuitively know to be false but that cling to me via ego—limiting beliefs about my abilities or my worthiness—and the first step in shifting and healing anything is awareness.

DREAM JOURNALING SELF-REFLECTION RITUAL

This kind of self-reflection is valuable with any kind of journaling, but with dream journaling it is truly about tapping into your deepest wells of inner knowing because the messages coded into your dreams are coming only from within.

You Will Need:

- Your dream journal with at least one week of dreams recorded in it
- Pen or pencil
- White candle
- Diluted lavender essential oil

Light the candle. Sit in front of it in a comfortable position and close your eyes for a moment. Take a deep, cleansing breath and release it with a sigh.

Sigh out anything that feels heavy and unsupportive in this moment and allow your mind to clear. Drop your shoulders away from your ears and relax deeply into your body.

Rub a little lavender essential oil on your fingertips and anoint the place on your forehead just above and between your closed eyes. Rub the oil onto your skin in a clockwise motion, to allow in positive energy and to open your third eye, the gateway to your intuition.

When you're ready, open your eyes and open your dream journal. Read through as many dreams as you like. You can read through them in order, from beginning to end, read a particular period of time, or simply skim through and read any that call to you.

On the next blank page of your journal or on a blank piece of paper, write down any thoughts that come up as you are reading. Especially look for themes that come up repeatedly, whether they be recurring struggles you've faced, common symbols or images you seem to see frequently in your dreams, or anything else that catches your attention.

When you have finished reading, look over your notes. What emerges? What coded messages have been appearing in your dreams over the period that you've read?

How has your intuition been speaking through your dreams in the big picture?

What are the next steps you are meant to take?

Answer these questions and any others you find on your heart in your journal. When you feel complete, blow out the candle.

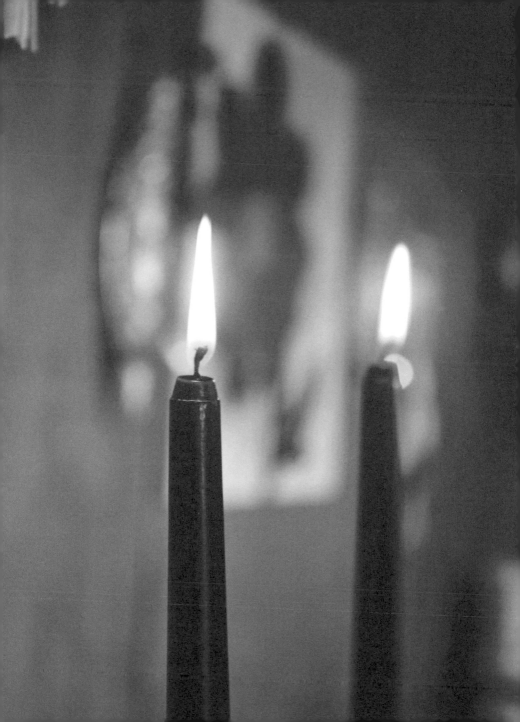

Scrying: A Direct Line to Your Higher Self

There are many different forms of divination. You can read tea leaves. You can practice bibliomancy, the practice of reading a passage in a book at random and drawing meaning from it. You can read tarot cards.

But perhaps one of the most mysterious and witchy forms of divination is scrying. Scrying is essentially the act of gazing into something (usually a mirror, a crystal, or a candle flame), in order to ascertain the answer to a question. This might sound highly esoteric and inaccessible but if you've ever stared into the flickering flames of the fireplace or a campfire, then you've pretty much practiced scrying.

The basic principle of scrying is disassociation. You're giving the conscious mind something physical to focus on so that you can access your intuition and your higher self without ego or conscious thought getting in the way.

Like all forms of divination, scrying offers an opportunity for self-reflection. Most of all, scrying allows you to truly ask for guidance directly from your intuition. I love scrying for the way that it opens a direct connection to my intuition without the influence of outside perspectives. Scrying is basically like picking up the phone and calling your higher self.

CANDLE SCRYING RITUAL

Though you can practice this same technique by gazing into a clear crystal ball or a mirror, candle scrying is my personal favorite variation because it's so easily accessible. Crystal balls can be expensive (though aesthetically, *very* witchy), and I find gazing into my own reflection more distracting than enlightening. But gazing into a flame, even a tiny candle flame, awakens something deeply primal within you. Humans have probably been staring into the depths of fire since we discovered this life-sustaining force millennia ago.

You Will Need:

- Taper candle (ideally black, as it allows you to focus on the flame as the only bright spot in your vision, but white will work as well)
- Small mirror (optional)

Place the candle in a safe holder and set it on your altar or a table that you can sit comfortably at. If you'd like to use the mirror too, you can prop it up behind the candle so that you can see the flame reflected in it but preferably not your own face.

Light the candle.

Turn off all the lights and make the room as dark as you can safely (draw the curtains, etc.).

Sit in front of the candle. You might fold your arms on the table or place your forearms flat on either side of the candle holder.

Close your eyes and take a few deep, cleansing breaths. Take a moment to clear your mind as much as you can to ground yourself.

Open your eyes and gaze softly at the candle flame. Breathe softly, if it is comfortable to do so, so as not to disturb the flame too much.

Gaze into the heart of the flame and allow your mind to expand. Allow your eyes to become unfocused.

You may ask a specific question but I often find that scrying is most effective when you just let your mind wander. Your intuition will guide you to the thoughts and ideas that you are meant to have.

Allow the messages and images that come to you to enter your mind, to float through your consciousness, and then let them drift away. Anything you are meant to carry with you out of this practice will stay with you.

When you're ready, refocus your eyes and allow your breath to deepen again. Come back into your body.

Blow out the candle.

You may want to do some journaling about the messages that have come up for you during your session.

Chapter 9
SELF-CARE RITUALS FOR GETTING BACK TO NATURE

Feeling connected to nature is one of the number one reasons why people pursue a spiritual path, especially as a witch. Witchcraft is inherently linked to the natural world and the cycles of nature. Our celebrations honor the movement of the sun and moon and the passing of the seasons. Our tools almost exclusively come from nature, whether they be dried herbs, crystals, or essential oils. Witches care deeply about the earth and the environment. And the archetype of the witch is also that of the wild woman, of the tree spirit, or forest dweller.

Yet most of us don't actually dwell in the forest. We don't live in cottages with thatched roofs and cauldrons on the hearth. We live in apartments and townhouses with tiny balconies and little privacy. We have windowsill gardens and concrete patios. We live surrounded by cement and yearn for fresh air and open spaces.

Feeling that connection to nature that awakens something primal within you is truly a form of self-care. Spending time in nature is ideal, of course, and if you are able to go for hikes regularly, to go kayaking, or just to go to the beach and put your toes in the sand, then do that. It can be hard though. Like most forms of self-care, it's something we think of as a luxury, as a leisure time activity. When life gets in the way, those recreational outdoor activities are some of the first things to go.

To be honest with you, I live close to about a dozen state parks and am only about forty minutes from the ocean, but I think I've been hiking once this year and to the beach maybe half a dozen times. Even proximity isn't always enough to overcome our many excuses and the guilt of taking time for ourselves.

The following self-care rituals are designed to help you get back to nature, even if you can't really get out in nature all that much. Some of these rituals make use of public green spaces or your own narrow patch of earth (or even concrete), but most of them take advantage of the natural tools of the witch as a connection to nature instead. Working with plants in all their forms (fresh, dried, oil, incense) is a great way to feel connected to the seasons and in flow with the natural rhythm of the universe. Drinking a cup of tea and diffusing a favorite essential oil are actually very intimate experiences of nature, bringing your mind and body into direct contact with the plants these tools are made from.

It might not always seem like it in the concrete jungle, but nature actually is all around. It's in the dandelions poking up through the sidewalk. It's there in the tree changing its leaves outside your office window. Awaken that primal connection to Mother Earth and get back to nature, for all its benefits of peace and awareness and to soothe your soul, with the following ritual ideas.

The Self-Care Wheel of the Year

I think the seasons are always an ideal place to start when talking about the rhythms of nature. The seasons impact us in such profound and undeniable ways, and yet their direct effect in our modern lives can sometimes be so subtle we miss it completely. With our electric lights and HVAC systems, we don't feel the changing of the seasons in the way that our ancient (or even fairly recent) ancestors did. We don't notice the days getting shorter and darker in the same way. Thankfully, most of us don't have to worry about having enough food to make it through the cold of winter.

Now, I'm not here to bemoan modern conveniences, but we do have to recognize the incredibly fast shift in the way that we interact with the seasons. Only a few generations ago, the cold and dark of winter and the heat of summer were inalienable facts of life that greatly impacted our ability to simply survive. Now, after only little more than a century, we've almost completely lost that innate connection to the passing of the seasons.

Thankfully, modern witches are reclaiming that connection and reclaiming the ancient festivals that celebrated the seasons. There is documentation of solstice and equinox celebrations all around the world throughout history. The Winter Solstice was alternately celebrated in the Celtic isles as Yule, in Scandinavia as Jul, and in ancient Rome as Saturnalia, not to mention the monuments that directly line up with the sun on the solstices, such as Newgrange in Ireland. Modern Wiccans and witches have reclaimed these ancient festivals and as much of the lore and history as we can in order to recapture the magick that comes when we are truly in flow with the natural rhythms of the universe.

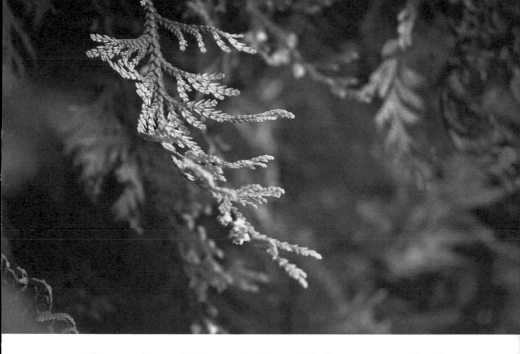

When we flow with those rhythms, with the seasons, and with the astrological movement of the sun and the planets, we can honor and nurture each of our own needs more deeply in their natural season. Winter is for rest and honoring the needs of the mind. Spring is for pleasure and honoring the needs of the body. Summer is for fun and honoring the primal need to connect with nature. Autumn is for gratitude and honoring the needs of your intuition and higher self.

The Wiccan Wheel of the Year is what most modern witches follow, at least to some degree. The Wheel consists of eight seasonal holidays (or "sabbats"), four of which are the solstices and equinoxes. The other four festivals equally divide the time between each solstice and equinox and are collectively known as the "fire festivals."

Many witches consider Samhain, the October 31 celebration

of the ancestors and the ancient predecessor to Halloween, to be the Witches' New Year, making it both the beginning and the end of the Wheel of the Year. During the season of Samhain, we honor the ancestors and all that has come before us, as well as practicing divination and intuitive work. Samhain is an ideal time for practicing shadow work and divination for nurturing your intuition.

After this magickal and auspicious celebration is the Winter Solstice, which occurs each year on December 20–22 when the sun reaches 0° of Capricorn. As the longest night of the year, the Winter Solstice is a celebration of both embracing the dark and lighting it up with our joy—and with literal lights, which is why we decorate trees and our homes with lights and candles at this time of year. It is an ideal time to really honor your need for rest and retreat.

Next up is Imbolc, the fire festival that occurs on February 1. Imbolc is the sabbat perhaps most directly linked to self-care as it is all about resting before spring comes and nurturing your needs.

The Spring Equinox on March 20–22, when the sun reaches 0° of Aries, ushers in a new season. Also in the spring season, on May 1, is Beltane or May Day, the ancient festival of fertility and abundance. The equinox and Beltane are celebrated with eggs, flowers, and symbols of the earth's fertility, making it an ideal time to create what you really want in your life and to honor your sensual, physical needs.

The Summer Solstice occurs on June 20–22 when the sun reaches 0° of Cancer, and is the longest day of the year, when the sun reaches its peak. The solstice is truly a day of celebration and fun, of spending time outside and nurturing your primal connection to nature.

As the sun begins to wind down, the last two sabbats of the year carry us into autumn. Lammas, the first harvest festival, takes place on August 1 and is the first harbinger of the end of summer. It is a bountiful celebration of the summer harvest. The Autumn Equinox occurs on September 20–22 when the sun reaches 0° of Libra, and is known as the Witches' Thanksgiving. Both Lammas and the equinox are about celebrating and expressing gratitude for all that we have been blessed with, making it the perfect time to break bread with loved ones and recommit to your greatest devotions.

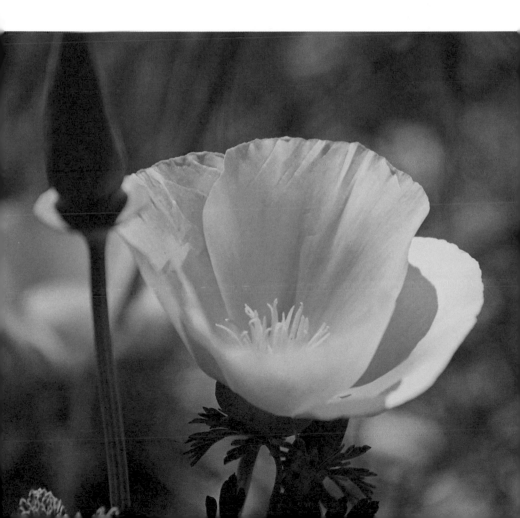

Essential Oil Blends for the Four Seasons

There are many ways to celebrate the seasons and these eight festivals, most of them directly connected to the plants that are in season during that time. Although in today's world, we import fruits and veggies and even flowers from other countries when they aren't in season in our own, there was a time not so very long ago when plants were only available when they were actually in season. While it's theoretically great to be able to have citrus in summer and tomatoes in winter, there's nothing like eating with the seasons when fruits and veggies are each at their ripest, juiciest peak.

While many of us have well-stocked essential oil collections that span the seasons, using oils that align with the naturally in-season plants as well is a great way to fill your home with the scent of the season. The following four essential oil blends are perfect for diffusing at the solstices and equinoxes and all through each of the seasons that follow them to help you align with the natural energies throughout the year:

SPRING EQUINOX ESSENTIAL OIL BLEND

- 5 drops lemon oil
- 3 drops lavender oil
- 2 drops rose oil

SUMMER SOLSTICE ESSENTIAL OIL BLEND

- 5 drops geranium oil
- 3 drops rosemary oil
- 2 drops oregano oil

AUTUMN EQUINOX ESSENTIAL OIL BLEND

- 5 drops patchouli oil
- 3 drops angelica oil
- 2 drops sage oil

WINTER SOLSTICE ESSENTIAL OIL BLEND

- 4 drops pine oil
- 3 drops cedarwood oil
- 2 drops cinnamon oil
- 2 drops clove oil
- 2 drops nutmeg oil

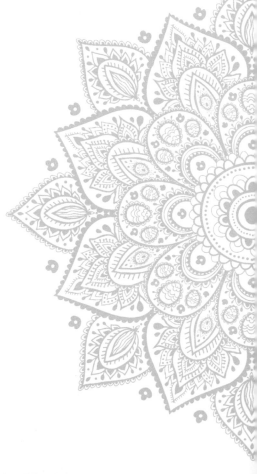

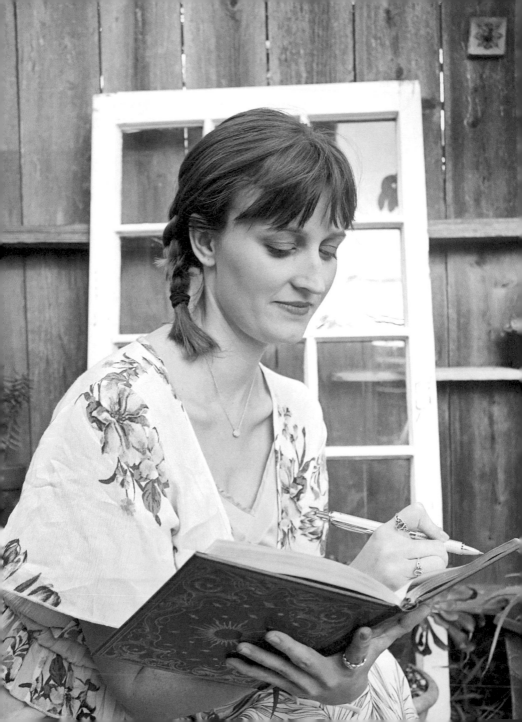

City Park Meditation with Seasonal Nature Journaling

Even if you don't have a patch of earth to truly call your own, you can still meditate and spend time in nature by making use of city parks and public green spaces. Most modern cities have at least some kind of small public park that you can visit for this ritual.

Visiting the same park again and again, throughout the seasons, is a great way to really tune in to the rhythms of nature. It's one thing to notice the seasons as they arrive, once most of the trees have turned orange in autumn or flowers are blooming everywhere in spring. But paying close attention to one place will allow you to see the subtle shifts—the harbingers of each season in the months prior to their actual arrival.

You Will Need:

- Journal and pen
- Picnic blanket (optional)

You'll want a comfortable place to sit so either bring a blanket with you to spread on the grass or find a safe, quiet bench to sit on. This is also a great opportunity to exercise outdoors, whether you bring your yoga mat with you to practice asanas on the grass or go for a run in the park before your meditation.

Find your seat and get comfy. I recommend choosing a spot where you can easily see at least a couple of trees and other plants, whether they are wild or landscaped, as well as somewhere the sun will not be in your eyes. You'll be returning to this same spot each time you want to practice this ritual. If it's noisy in the park, you might want to put headphones in with instrumental music, but try to find a quiet enough spot where you can listen to the birds and the breeze instead.

Begin by closing your eyes and taking a deep breath of fresh air. Inhale through your nose and exhale through your mouth, sighing out loud. Place your hands on your knees and drop your shoulders away from your ears, grounding into the earth.

When you're ready, open your eyes. This is a different kind of meditation than you might be used to. In this case, you aren't trying to tune out and clear your mind completely. Rather, this is a waking meditation, if you will, where the goal is to tune *in* to the world around you.

Find a focal point to focus your eyes on, right at the ground level. Survey the earth. What is the ground composed of (dirt, grass, bark)? Is it flat or uneven? Is there evidence of people or animals there?

When you're ready, lift your eyes to the plants growing in this same spot. What kinds of plants are here? What stage of life are they in at the moment (new growth, buds, blooming, drooping, broken leaves or branches, dying)?

Next, lift your eyes to any nearby trees. What kinds of trees are here? Are they evergreens, deciduous, or coniferous? What kind of condition are they in (full and lush, overgrown, dying)? How are the seasons affecting them—are they blooming, losing their leaves, bare? Can you spot any birds or creatures?

Finally, lift your eyes to the sky. What does the sky look like today? What shade of blue is it right now? Are there clouds? If so, what do they look like (white and puffy, gray and threatening, wispy)? Can you see any images or intuitive messages in the clouds?

Slowly bring your eyes back down from the sky, over the tops of the trees, down the tree trunks, into the plants, and settle back on the earth. Take a deep breath in through your nose and exhale through your mouth.

In your journal, write down anything you noticed in particular about the ground, plants, trees, or sky and date the entry. How can you see evidence of the current season in this green space?

Ideally, practice this meditation and journaling exercise at least once a month or even as often as once a week. The more frequently you do this in the same spot, the more you'll start to notice the subtle shifts and the more aware you'll become of the natural rhythms of the universe.

Depending on your schedule and availability, you might also consider practicing weekly nature journaling about a scene you can access more easily, such as the scene out your bedroom or office window, and practice the city park meditation less frequently.

Working with Native Plants & Herbs

Some plants have become utterly passé and expected within the spiritual community, such as sage and patchouli. Unfortunately, many of these plants are directly impacted by cultural appropriation and spiritual bypassing. White sage, in particular, is sacred to many Native American tribes and has been heavily harvested due to its popularity as a "spiritual" herb. White sage is burned to clear bad energy and negative spirits in a ritual called smudging. This term is actually specific to some Native American tribes and using the term without a deep understanding of the ritual in its original context is straight-up cultural appropriation. However, cleansing with smoke from various plants is a common practice throughout the Americas, Europe, and Asia.

It's important to understand the origins and traditions of the actual rituals you choose to practice and why they are sacred to those who practice them. It is all too easy to purchase something online or in a shop without having a deep understanding of why it is sacred, which is why it is so important to learn about working with plants and herbs that are native either to your local area or to your own ancestral cultures. As we become more and more aware of the global impact of colonization and cultural appropriation, making sure you are aligned with your spiritual and ethical values is definitely a form of self-care.

Learning about plants that are native to your own area can be a lot of fun. When you become aware of the plants that grow naturally around you, you'll start to spot them everywhere. My favorite resource for my own area is the *Sunset Western Garden Book*. Similar publications have been written about many different regions, but

I recommend simply starting with an Internet search or visiting a local nursery to inquire in person about native plants.

Once you know what plants are growing around you, you can work directly with them as replacements for over-harvested herbs. For example, if cedar is in abundance near you, you can use a locally harvested option as an excellent cleansing plant to burn instead of white sage. You'll want to research the metaphysical and magickal properties of the native plants you discover. I recommend starting with *Cunningham's Encyclopedia of Magical Herbs* to learn about the spiritual energy of many common plants.

Learning about plants that are native to your ancestral cultures, especially those used for spiritual rituals, can be even more powerful and eye-opening. Pretty much every culture has used plants in rituals in one form or another, whether it be as burnt offerings, incense, tea, or even in specially prepared foods. Resources for this journey of discovery will depend entirely on the cultures that your ancestors hailed from but I encourage you to dig deep with this. Working with plants that were likely used by your own ancestors many generations ago (and having an awareness of that connection) is a magickal experience I can't properly describe for you—you just have to experience it!

RITUAL TO CONNECT WITH THE ENERGY OF A PLANT

Whatever plants you connect with through your research, the following ritual will help you connect with each of them on a deep, spiritual level.

You Will Need:

- Your chosen plant (either a cutting or live plant)
- Additional forms of the plant, such as an oil (optional)
- Divination tool of your choosing
- Journal and pen

Lovingly place your chosen plant on your altar. If working with multiple forms of the plant, set up your tools as needed (such as begin diffusing the oil). Find a comfortable seat where you can see and touch the plant.

Place your hands on either side of the plant, not quite touching it, and close your eyes. Take a deep breath in and exhale out loud, relaxing deeply into your body.

Imagine that the plant begins to glow between your hands, its energy and spirit surrounding it in an aura. The energy begins to expand and permeate your hands. You can feel the warmth of its glow. The plant's energy rises up your arms and down through your entire body, until you are fully connected to it.

When you are ready, open your eyes and pick the plant up in your hands. Feel its texture, smell it.

Reach for the divination tool of your choosing. Ask the plant what messages it has for you and use your tools to receive that message. (For example, you might draw a tarot card to help you.)

Record the intuitive message you receive in your journal and anything else you feel is important to recall about the plant.

Keep the plant on your altar for as long as you wish and return to it again and again to dig deeper and receive additional messages from it.

Repeat this ritual with every plant you wish to work with.

Green Witch Tea Ritual & Recipe

One thing that I find *almost* universal among witches is a great love of tea. There is just something innately magickal about steeping plants in hot water and then sipping a cozy and healing cup of tea.

No matter the season, no matter the mood, there's always a cup of tea for that.

In fact, tea herbalism is a pillar of my own spiritual practice and is a key element of how I connect with nature. Whether I'm steeping a blend of my own making, a blend I purchased from a favorite shop, or combining herbs right in my cup, working with plants and tea leaves is how this cottage witch channels the energy of nature from the comfort of my cozy suburban townhouse.

This particular tea ritual and recipe are inspired by the path of the green witch, the earthiest and most grounded of the paths. The green witch honors nature in all its forms (wild, tamed, healing, poisonous), and loves to get her hands in the dirt. If that sounds like you, or if you just wish to connect with earth energy through the power of tea, then try out this blend for yourself.

If you are able to use any of these herbs from your own garden, definitely do that—otherwise, store-bought will be just fine.

I was first exposed to this kind of tea on a trip to Amsterdam, where mint tea is a native favorite. It seemed like every café offered fresh mint tea which was really just a clear glass mug stuffed with fresh mint leaves and hot water poured over the top. After a few glasses of this refreshingly cozy beverage, I was completely sold. A recipe like this is about as close to nature as you can get from the comfort of your couch!

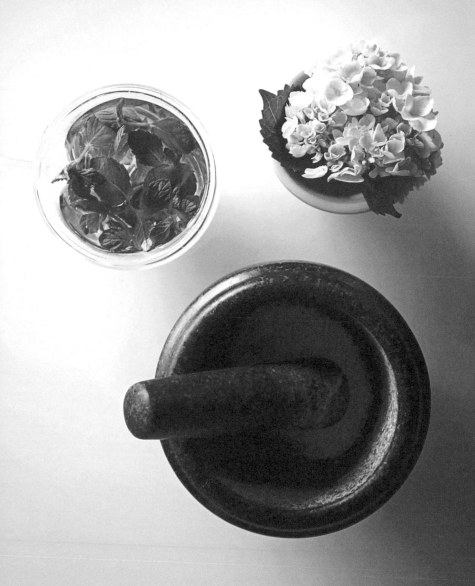

Fun Fact: This kind of "tea" made only with herbs and no actual tea leaves, which come from the Camellia sinensis plant, is actually called a "tisane."

Ingredients:

- Fresh, organic mint leaves
- Fresh, organic lemon verbena leaves
- Fresh, organic chamomile flowers
- Optional: any other herbs you wish to include!

Rinse all of the herbs you wish to include and pat dry with a towel.

Picking up each bundle, rub the herbs between your hands to release their scent. Lift them to your face and inhale their healing aroma. Notice the distinct differences and commonalities between each.

You might say a small prayer here to express your gratitude to the plant itself or to Mother Nature for providing this plant to nourish and soothe you.

Place the herbs directly in your mug. (A clear glass mug works very nicely for this so you can see all of the herbs but is not necessary.)

Pour hot water over the herbs and allow to steep at least five minutes before drinking.

Container Garden Blessing & Protection Spell

A garden blessing is one of the quintessential spells to cast for new witches. Blessing your home or garden space is a positive and uplifting way to practice a little magick and bring love and light into your sphere. There are almost endless ways to cast blessing spells. Personally, I like to infuse a blessing with protective energy to safeguard and extend the positivity that the spell brings to a space.

If you live in a small apartment or somewhere with little to no outdoor space, you might think that a garden blessing isn't applicable to you, but that's where the beauty of container gardening comes in!

Container gardens, gardening in pots on a patio or even windowsill, are an excellent solution for small-space gardening needs. They're perfect for the witch who wants to grow her own herbs but doesn't have a full garden of her own.

This spell is designed especially for those working with container gardens but can be easily adapted to bless and protect any garden space!

One of the oldest spells that we have actual physical evidence of is called a "witch bottle." Witch bottles are often dug up in foundations or yards of homes that were built in the sixteenth, seventeenth, and eighteenth centuries in the Americas and Britain.

A witch bottle is essentially a glass jar filled with a variety of objects (often sharp, pointy objects for protection and some kind of acid or honey for binding), and then buried, usually near the front door of the home or placed in the foundation during building.

Container gardens offer the perfect opportunity for a modern witch bottle, as it's easy to bury a small jar in a pot, regardless of where it is.

You Will Need:

- Black, white, or green candle
- Wax paper
- Small glass jar, such as a 5-ounce mason jar
- Sage or cedar bundle for cleansing
- Safety pins for protection
- Small green calcite crystal for nourishment and connecting to earth
- Small tiger's-eye crystal for protection and prosperity
- Oak leaves or acorns for fertility
- Salt for purification and protection
- Honey for binding and sweetness
- Soil
- Pot
- Plant

Light a candle in the color of your choosing (black for protection, white for blessing, or green for prosperity). Lay the wax paper out on your work surface.

Unscrew the lid from the jar. Light your sage or cedar bundle and pass the jar through the purifying smoke a few times to clear it of any existing energy. (Alternatively, you could spritz the jar with purifying essential oils.)

Open each of the safety pins and place them in the jar. Place each of the crystals and leaves or acorns in the jar. Sprinkle in the salt.

Fill the jar about half full of honey, just until all of the objects are covered. Screw the lid on tightly.

Blow out the candle and lift it carefully. Holding the jar over the wax paper, drip candle wax around the outside of the lid to seal it.

Once the wax has dried, scoop a bit of soil into the bottom of the pot. Place the jar in the pot and cover over with soil. Proceed to plant and water the live plant. Place the pot near to the entrance of your garden area to bless and protect the surroundings.

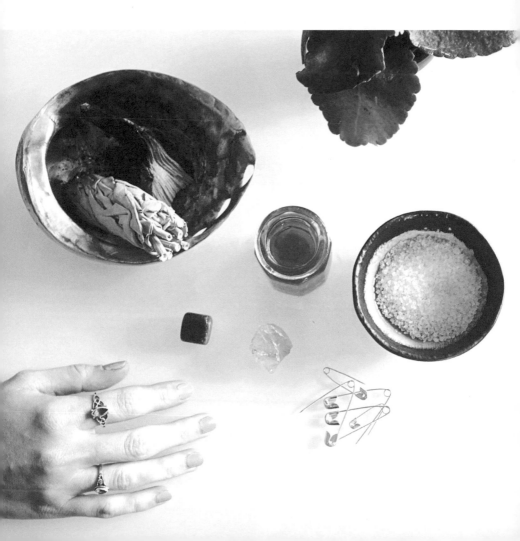

Chapter 10
SELF-CARE RITUALS FOR DISCOVERING DEVOTION

Devotion is the heart and soul of self-care. Without devotion to something or someone, we drift aimlessly through life.

A major part of practicing soulful, spiritual self-care is expressing your love for the things you care about most. If those soul-level people and causes aren't an active part of your daily experience, you're going to experience that lost, aimless drifting instead. You're going to feel unfulfilled, even if you're doing all the intuitive work and taking care of your mind and body and connecting with nature and getting intimate with your astrological chart.

All the other elements of self-care that I've introduced in this book are pieces of the puzzle that is completed by discovering devotion in your life. Devotion brings it all home and gives you focus for every ritual and every act of self-care.

Devotion can be to yourself, to a person, a group of people, a deity, a cause, or to the rhythms of the universe. We can pretty much categorize these as an internal or external expression of devotion.

Internal expressions of devotion are the very definition of self-love, of choosing to dedicate yourself to your highest potential and to being kind and gentle with yourself. Shadow work, expressing your creativity, and being healthy are all examples of internal devotion.

External expressions of devotion include the traditional definitions of being devoted to a romantic partner or to a god or goddess, as well as devotion to your family, to a political ideal, or even to your ancestors. Anything you are devoted to outside of yourself is an externally expressed devotion.

The rhythms of the universe, including the moon phases, astrological transits, and the seasons, are sort of like a subset of external devotion, if you will. The universal rhythms are their own category because, while they are obviously external, you are also one with them in a way: as above, so below. The way that the stars and planets move through the sky or the way that you experience each of the seasons impacts you in a unique way and many witches choose to express devotion to one or more of these rhythmic cycles for that reason.

Most likely, you have certain internal *and* external expressions of devotion in your life, though there are likely one or two things that you are most focused on.

The ideas and rituals on the following pages are designed to inspire you to really think about what does light you up, what you are most devoted to. What cause or person or idea do you believe in with your whole soul? What do you feel incomplete without?

With all the tools and magick in this book, you are well-equipped to create self-care rituals that nourish your soul and nurture your inner witch—just remember to always allow the wisdom of your intuition and the spark of devotion to guide you, and your spiritual self-care practice will sustain you through whatever comes your way.

Self-Love Altar

Self-care is the real-world expression of self-love. When you are empowered to love all aspects of yourself, you are honoring the divine within. Self-care is how you express the *fact* that the divine masculine and divine feminine reside within you and you deserve to be treated as such.

Setting up a self-love altar is an excellent way to ground your inner divinity in reality. Altars are one of my favorite ways to focus and direct energy, as they are easy (and fun!) to create and are a constant reminder of your intentions or devotion.

Set up your self-love altar anywhere that you'll see it on a daily basis. Some great locations include on your vanity or bathroom counter, somewhere private but with easy, regular access. You can include pretty much anything that brings you joy in your self-love altar but here are a few ideas to get you started:

- A mirror
- Handwritten poems or quotes
- Your favorite printed photos of yourself
- Crystals such as rose quartz, rose opal, raw emerald, desert rose
- Small potted plants such as mini tea roses or your favorite herb
- Rose-scented sachets, sprays, or candles
- Figurine of the goddess Venus, Aphrodite, or Kuan Yin

Use your altar as a place of safety and sanctuary. During your day-to-day, when you are simply passing by it in your busy life, your self-love altar is there to serve as a reminder of your devotion to loving your body, being kind to yourself, and nourishing all of your needs. However, it is also a sacred space that you've created as a magickal place to recharge your batteries.

Try setting aside an hour or two every week to sit at your altar, journal, read cards, or just read a book. This space is sacred because it is the grounded, real-world expression of your choice to love yourself.

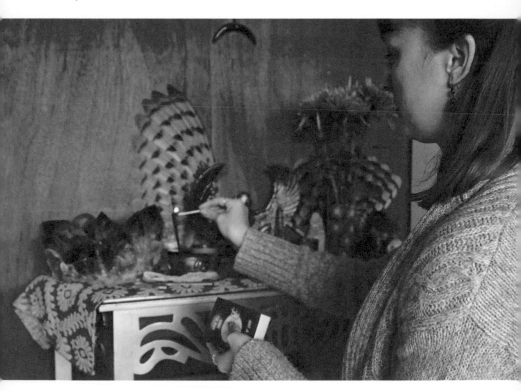

Shadow Work Journaling Ritual

Shadow work is one of the most important ingredients in your self-care cauldron. The shadow self, or shadow aspect, is the part of you that you push down, push away, bury deep inside. It's anything that makes you feel shame, fear, or doubt. Doing shadow work is the process of becoming aware of those feelings, acknowledging and understanding them, and then transmuting them into something more positive, productive, or even a strength.

We all carry around social programming, limiting beliefs, and negative self-talk that we may not even be fully conscious of. Often, we have deeply ingrained beliefs about who we are, what we can be, how we can express ourselves, and what we are capable of feeling or doing, beliefs that are embedded in our subconscious but have little to no foundation in reality.

Devotion to yourself can be expressed in many ways, of course, and shadow work is an excellent way to express devotion to your mental and emotional health. So much of being a witch is about awareness: awareness of the rhythms of the universe, awareness of your innate inner power and intuition, and, perhaps above all, self-awareness. Shadow work is one way to practice that self-awareness and to shed old beliefs that no longer serve your highest potential.

But what actually is shadow work, in a practical sense? A big part of it is meditation and journaling. Often, just knowing the right question to ask of yourself can be all you need to break down deeply embedded shadows.

You Will Need:

- Black candle, as black is the color of banishing

- Smoky quartz crystal for banishing
- Journal and pen
- Fire-safe container

Light the black candle.

Write down any "negative" feelings or beliefs that you hold about yourself or the world. For example, you might write down that you feel shame around expressing your sensuality or that you wish you would react less emotionally to certain situations.

Cup your hands around the smoky quartz crystal, which is great for banishing negativity and for opening your mind and heart to see your shadow self more clearly. Close your eyes and let your shoulders drop, focusing on the weight of the crystal in your hands. Think about the list of things you've just written down and allow one to float to the top naturally. Don't overthink this—whatever shadow comes up that you want to address is the one you are intuitively meant to work on in this ritual.

On a new page in your journal, journal on the following prompts:

- What is my earliest memory of having this feeling or belief?
- What would be possible if this belief were not true?
- What evidence can I find in my life or in the world to demonstrate that a new, more positive, and more supportive belief is true?

When you feel ready, write down the old belief or feeling that you've just been working with on a separate scrap of paper. Hold the paper to the candle flame and drop it into the fire-safe container to burn, banishing a layer of shadow from your life.

Art Magick Sketchbook Grimoire

For those with a creative spark (perhaps with a strong Leo or fifth house placement in their astrological chart), expressing your creativity through the art form that speaks to your soul is the ultimate form of devotion. Art can heal, art can uplift, and art can make us question everything we believe to be true. Art is powerful in so many ways and it becomes even more so when combined with a little magick.

The most important aspect of spellcasting is your will and intention—not any of the tools or trappings. However, as you've learned in this book, tools can help direct your energy with greater power and accuracy. Whether you are pointing a wand or sweeping paint onto a canvas, your tools of choice can help you to build energy around your intentions.

Art magick is exactly what it sounds like, casting spells and crafting rituals around your preferred art form, so if expressing yourself creatively is what you're most devoted to, then this ritual is for you.

You Will Need:

- The tools of your preferred visual art form (such as paint-brushes, pens, collage materials, or charcoal)
- Sketchbook

This ongoing ritual employs a blank sketchbook as a grimoire, a sacred book where a witch records her practice. Instead of (or in addition to) journaling each day, create a work of art that speaks to your intuitive wisdom and expresses your devotion to your creativity! You can incorporate written words into the pages that you decorate and use any materials that speak to you to create something beautiful and soulful. Turn this daily creative pursuit into a ritual itself or incorporate it into your morning or evening ritual.

You can adapt this to suit your own practice and beliefs in many different ways:

- Create an art page to record the mood and theme of your dreams each morning.
- Create an art page to record and respond to your daily tarot card reading.
- Create an art page to honor the new and full moons each month.
- Create an art page to honor different aspects of the deity you work with.

A sketchbook grimoire is not only a deeply personal way to express yourself, it's also a beautiful and healing record of your spiritual and self-care practice.

Kitchen Witch Morning Devotional

We've talked about what it means to be a green witch, so now I want to share more about one of the other more popular witchcraft paths: kitchen witchcraft. Being a kitchen witch means that the kitchen is the heart and soul of your spiritual practice. All or most of your spells are recipes and cooking and eating are devotional practices for you.

Practicing kitchen magick is a great way to express devotion in a variety of ways: you might be devoted to eating healthy, to making home-cooked meals for your family, or to consuming locally sourced foods. Whatever your reason, kitchen devotionals are an excellent way to integrate the magickal and the mundane in your life, which is a key component of developing a sustainable and supportive self-care practice.

Whether or not you consider yourself a "good" cook, we all gotta eat! The beauty of kitchen magick is that you can practice magick and express your spirituality, all while doing mundane daily tasks. Anytime you can combine your spiritual and self-care practice with something you're already doing, it's going to be that much easier to stick with it.

This morning devotional is a daily ritual you can incorporate into your morning routine to start the day off with a little magick.

You Will Need:

- Yogurt
- Seasonal berries or fruit
- Almonds or other nuts

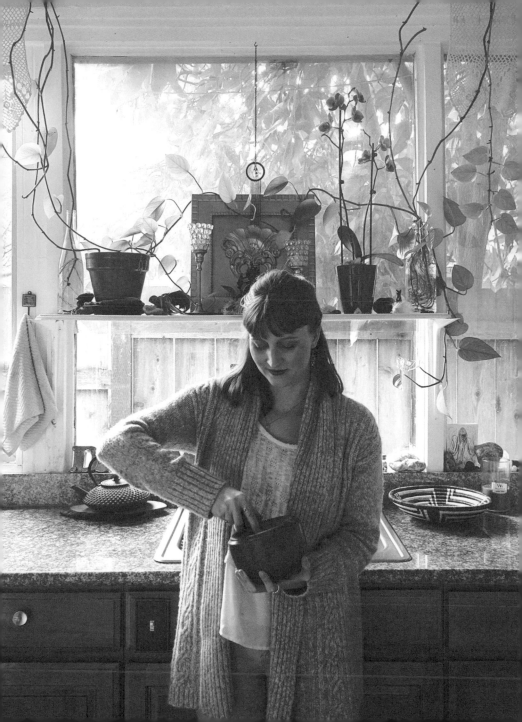

- Ground cinnamon (during new and waxing moon phases)
- Ground cardamom (during full and waning moon phases)
- Other favorite yogurt toppings, such as granola or dried fruit

Walk into the kitchen and begin your usual morning routine, but take a few moments standing at the counter to close your eyes, take a deep breath, and sigh it out. Even if it's just a couple seconds, even if everything around you is chaotic, just take this one breath to center yourself at the beginning of the day.

Scoop your yogurt into a bowl and sprinkle your favorite toppings on. This is a great opportunity to eat seasonally, using fresh berries and fruits. (My personal favorite yogurt bowl recipe is vanilla bean yogurt topped with blackberries, salted roasted almonds, and cinnamon.) Sprinkle ground cinnamon or ground cardamom over the bowl. You can align with the moon phases by using cinnamon, ruled by the element of fire, during new and waxing moon phases, and cardamom, ruled by the element of water, during full and waning moon phases, or find other spices you enjoy. Stir to combine the ingredients in your yogurt bowl with intention. If it is a new or waxing moon phase, stir the bowl *deosil* (clockwise) to call in good energy. If it is a full or waning moon phase, stir it *widdershins* (counterclockwise) to banish negativity from your day.

If you can, find a quiet moment to enjoy your breakfast and continue focusing on calling in the good or banishing the negative. You might put on a little music or a guided meditation or light some candles. Even if your morning is otherwise harried, though, it's okay. Incorporating even this little bit of magick into your morning will start you off on the right note.

Ancestor Veneration Ritual for Guidance

Ancestor veneration might sound like something shrouded in mystery but it's actually an easy and beautiful way to connect with your roots. Ancestors are honored in many cultures and have been important to personal and societal growth throughout history. Even today, many countries have rituals to venerate or honor the ancestors, including India, China, and Mexico. Honoring the ancestors is an important part of the celebrations that surround Samhain, the Celtic pagan sabbat that takes place on October 31.

Whenever we practice divination, meditate, or journal in search of answers, we are seeking guidance from something greater than ourselves. Where you believe that guidance actually comes from is entirely up to you. It could be from the concept of your higher self, a version of yourself that is free of ego and shadow and can lead you in the right direction. It could be from a god or goddess. It could be from your intuition or inner knowing (in which case you are seeking guidance from something great inside of yourself which is a powerful thing to think about). That guidance can also come from the ancestors. This idea of seeking guidance is a form of self-care in that it can be incredibly comforting. It's about trusting your guides to help you find the right path and knowing that you aren't in it all alone.

Working with your ancestors is also a powerful way to consciously fight against cultural appropriation in your own spiritual practice. Learning about your own ancestral cultures and roots can help you make more informed decisions about how you want to express your spirituality, rather than borrowing ideas from cultures that are not your own.

And, remember: if you have a difficult relationship with your own family, you can focus on your ancient pagan ancestors only.

If receiving wisdom from your ancestors is something that speaks to you, this ritual will help you listen for their guidance.

You Will Need:

- A family tree or photos of family members who have passed on (optional)
- Representations of your ancient ancestral cultures (such as figurines, fabrics, or amulets)
- Votive candles
- Your preferred divination tools

Create a little altar to your ancestors, using the family tree, photos, and/or representations of your ancient ancestral cultures. For example, you might have a photo of your great-grandmother and a printout of your family crest. This can be very inconspicuous—even a mantel with family photos can be an ancestor altar!

Each day, sit or stand at your ancestor altar and light the votive candle there. Take a few moments to ground and center yourself. Practice your daily divination ritual here, asking the ancestors for messages you need to receive for the day. See if any themes begin to emerge after a few days or weeks. The more you do this, the clearer the messages will become and you'll become more confident in knowing when it is your ancestors guiding you.

Extinguish the candle when you are finished.

Hex the Patriarchy Activism Ritual

"Hex the Patriarchy" became a fervent catchphrase of modern witches in the late 2010s, a cry for us all to combine our collective power and bring down the patriarchal status quo of the past through witchcraft. For many witches, justice is the ideal most worthy of expressing devotion for, with the political and social turmoil we find ourselves surrounded by.

There are endless political causes to devote your energy to, whether it be women's rights, LGBTQA rights, racial inequality, the environment, education, whatever most calls to your heart and soul, because politics are an inherently emotional endeavor.

The "Hex the Patriarchy" phrase is actually somewhat controversial, because some witches believes that you should never cast hexes or curses. Others believe that it is a privilege to choose not to use the powerful energy of intention and magick and that hexes and curses are sometimes our best tools for fighting injustice. Whatever you choose to believe is, as always, entirely up to you.

This particular ritual is not a hex but rather a way of focusing energy on what change you want to bring into the world. If your political beliefs are an important core of who you are, this ritual will help you express that passionate devotion in your spirituality while taking mindful action through magick.

You Will Need:

- Black candles
- Photo of a female politician or thought leader you admire
- Blank piece of paper
- String

- Tape
- Pen

Light the candles.

Tape the photo you've chosen to the center of the blank piece of paper. You might meditate for a few minutes on why you chose this particular person to represent the new movement.

Lay the string over the photo in a pentagram (a five-pointed star), taping it down at the corners. The pentagram represents the four elements and the concept of spirit. It is a sacred symbol of wholeness and a potent way to direct energy.

At each of the five corners of paper, write a shift you want to see and experience in the world.

Keep this pentagram on your altar or tuck it safely in your grimoire. Revisit it regularly to remind yourself of the shifts you are bringing into the world.

The Rhythms of the Universe

Many witches feel very in tune with the rhythms of the universe. In fact, our celebrations are inherently linked to the cycles of the moon phases, astrological transits, and the seasons. The seasonal sabbat celebrations each take place when the sun is in a particular astrological sign. The new moon is always in the same sign as the sun and the full moon is always in the opposite sign as the sun, and so all three of these universal cycles are intrinsically linked to one another.

HONORING THE MOON PHASES

The moon phases are often some of the first things that new witches experience in their practice. The idea of practicing a full moon ritual is an enticing one that evokes our sense of mystery and magick. Moon rituals are a great place to start because they're quite easy and

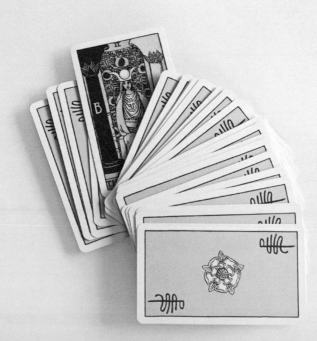

totally adaptable to your own needs so it's no surprise that so many of us start off here!

What are the moon phases and what makes them one of the rhythms of the universe?

It takes the moon approximately twenty-nine days to move through all twelve astrological signs and through all four phases.

The moon cycle begins at the new moon, when the moon is first invisible in the sky and then becomes the tiniest of slivers. The new moon always occurs in the same sign as the sun because the sun and moon are conjunct. Then, for about two weeks, the moon waxes toward full, growing larger and larger in the sky. It reaches its zenith with the beauty of the full moon, which is always in the sign opposite of the sun. Then the moon begins its descent again, waning back toward the new moon. Each phase is best suited to particular purposes:

- **New Moon:** Setting intentions, making plans
- **Waxing Moon:** Taking action, making moves
- **Full Moon:** Celebrating, aligning with intuition
- **Waning Moon:** Releasing, letting go

One of my favorite parts of the moon cycle is the fact that the full moon is always opposite the sun. There is so much balance and nourishing energy to be found on the full moon. The moon is ruled by the divine feminine and the sun is ruled by the divine masculine. The reason that we see the full face of the moon is because the sun is able to shine on it completely. We need both the masculine and the feminine to see the whole picture. Plus, since the sun and moon are in opposite signs on the full moon, it's as if the universe is giving us an opportunity to integrate a little more balance into our lives on that day.

The sun spends about a month in each astrological sign, while the moon only spends about two and a half days in each. So, for example, during Capricorn season we experience the sun in Capricorn for a month and all the energy of the divine masculine, of the desire for structure and responsibility, but then at some point during the season we also experience the full moon in Cancer, an opportunity to experience the lush, nurturing divine feminine energy that helps us balance out the strength of Capricorn. This happens in every season, a little gift of balance from the universe.

Many witches choose to do monthly new and/or full moon rituals or even a weekly ritual on the new, waxing quarter, full, and waning quarter moons. Following the lunar cycle is an excellent way to bring devotion into your spiritual and self-care practice because it provides such a regular rhythm to check in with yourself, your intuition, and the universe.

HONORING THE ASTROLOGICAL CYCLES

Following the astrological cycles is very similar to the moon phases but it represents a year-long cycle instead of a month-long one. As I mentioned, the sun spends about a month in each astrological sign, so it takes one year to pass through all twelve signs. Each sign represents a particular astrological season, when the sun is lighting up the energies of that sign and its highest expression:

- Aries: March/April
- Taurus: April/May

- Gemini: May/June
- Cancer: June/July
- Leo: July/August
- Virgo: August/September
- Libra: September/October
- Scorpio: October/November
- Sagittarius: November/December
- Capricorn: December/January
- Aquarius: January/February
- Pisces: February/March

The sun also moves around your own astrological chart throughout the year, lighting up each sign in your chart and reminding you of the values and virtues of each sign. For example, I have Leo in my twelfth house so when the sun is in Leo each year from late July to late August, it's lighting up the energies of my twelfth house, the house of dreams and imagination.

There are lots of ways to devote yourself to honoring the astrological seasons. You could have a sun altar that you ritually decorate each month or follow the sun around your own chart to tune into how the astrological cycles impact you personally, as described in Chapter 6 on page 130.

HONORING THE SEASONS

However, my favorite way to honor the astrological cycles is to also honor the seasons. As I shared in Chapter 9 on page 188, the seasonal sabbat celebrations of the pagan Wheel of the Year each align with a particular astrological sign. The solstices and equinoxes in particular occur at 0° of one of the cardinal signs of Aries, Cancer, Libra, and Capricorn.

You can think of your sabbat rituals, if you choose to do them, as astrological rituals as well. Rituals to honor the eight pagan sabbats are truly celebrations: celebrations of the movement of the sun through the sky and through the twelve signs. These festive occasions are typically honored with seasonal food and drink, dancing, music, and bonfires.

It's not required to celebrate the seasons astrologically, though. The changing sunlight, weather, and mood are also hallmarks of the passing seasons, of course. Our needs shift and evolve with the seasons, giving us renewed energy or a desire to rest and retreat. Honoring those shifts in your spiritual and self-care practice will help you to stay on track and nurture your needs through the ebbs and flows of life.

When I first began my own path as a witch almost a decade ago, I started by honoring the full moon—much as I had always done, looking up at the sky and being awed by the moon, whatever its phase. I quickly also began celebrating the seasonal sabbats, my first sabbat ritual having been for Lammas, the first harvest festival in August. It was some years later before I really discovered the magick of astrology and how the three cycles of the moon, seasons, and astrology are so inseparable from one another, but I was not at all surprised to discover that they are.

These universal rhythms are the foundation of my own devotion and of the magick that I practice. Above all, they provide weekly, monthly, and yearly checkpoints to ask myself: How can I nurture myself a little more deeply and with greater intention?

About the Author

Tenae Stewart is a practicing cottage witch and a self-love and empowerment coach. She is on a mission to bring the potent power of witchcraft into mainstream spiritual and wellness culture and to empower modern women to discover their inner witch! Tenae believes that witchcraft should be simple and empowering and her brand, The Witch of Lupine Hollow, is all about embodying simplicity in magick, ritual, and self-love practices.

She has spent nearly a decade studying and learning about magick, the moon phases, the seasons, and astrology and using these tools to develop rituals that resonate deeply with her. She loves sharing her experience and knowledge with others and helping them to take action to experience spiritual connection in their own real, daily lives.

Based in Northern California's Wine Country region, Tenae enjoys stargazing, rewatching *Practical Magic* and *Buffy the Vampire Slayer*, drinking rosé, and saying, "Wow, babe, look at the moon!" to her boyfriend every time she sees the moon, no matter what phase it's in. She's also an avid traveler and loves visiting new places; some of her favorite travel spots include Salem, Massachusetts, Savannah, Georgia, and Edinburgh, Scotland.

Tenae has been featured on a number of spiritual and witchy podcasts, including *I AM Goddess Collective*, a top-rated show on Apple Podcasts, and in articles on the popular lifestyle website Refinery29. Thousands of modern witches enjoy connecting with and learning from Tenae daily on her website, social media accounts, and free Facebook group.